the real skinny *on losing it*

the real skinny

skinny

on losing it

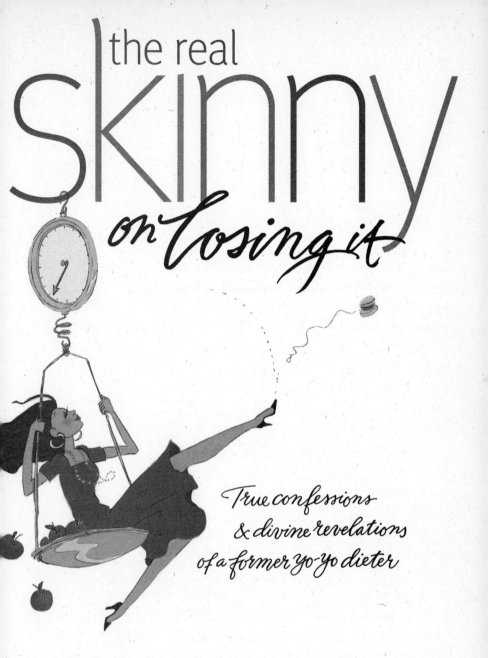

*True confessions
& divine revelations
of a former yo-yo dieter*

michelle mckinney hammond

Tyndale House Publishers, Inc., Carol Stream, Illinois

Visit Tyndale's exciting Web site at www.tyndale.com.

Visit Michelle McKinney Hammond at her Web site, www.michellehammond.com.

TYNDALE and Tyndale's quill logo are registered trademarks of Tyndale House Publishers, Inc.

The Real Skinny on Losing It: True Confessions and Divine Revelations of a Former Yo-Yo Dieter

Designed by Jennifer Ghionzoli

Edited by Katara Washington Patton

Published in association with the literary agency of Alive Communications, Inc., 7680 Goddard Street, Suite 200, Colorado Springs, CO 80920, www.alivecommunications.com.

Library of Congress Cataloging-in-Publication Data

McKinney Hammond, Michelle, date.
   The real skinny on losing it : true confessions and divine revelations of a former yo-yo dieter / Michelle McKinney Hammond.
      p. cm.
   Includes bibliographical references.
   ISBN 978-1-4143-3383-0 (sc)
1. Christian women—Religious life. 2. Self-perception in women—Religious aspects.
3. Reducing diets. I. Title. II. Title: True confessions and divine revelations of a former yo-yo dieter.
   BV4527.M423 2010
   248.8′43—dc22   2010036327

Printed in the United States of America

16   15   14   13   12   11   10
 7   6   5   4   3   2   1

contents

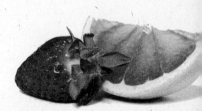

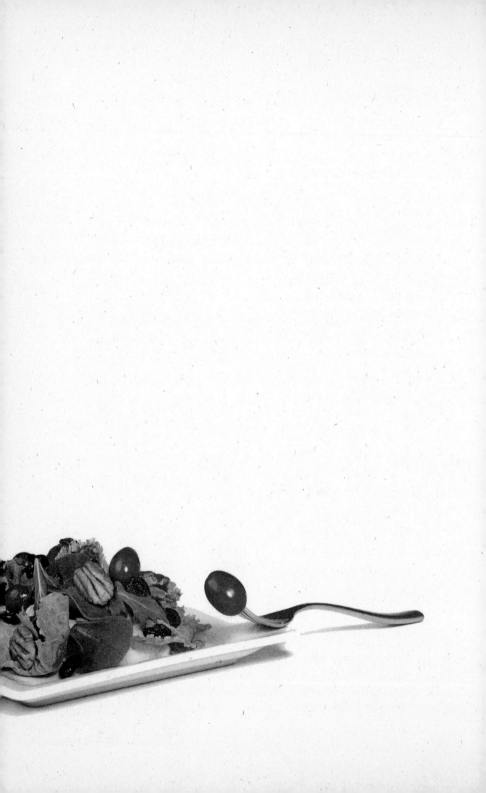

acknowledgments

To all those who love food as much as I do and more . . .

Ah well, here's to making a peace treaty with our hips and our lips. Ladies, pass the salad, please, and lift a water toast to totally losing it and living to see the dream of a svelter you come to life!

Carol Traver, I haven't decided if I should hug you or get you for sending me on this journey. ☺ Katara Patton, you are a bad mamma jamma. Thanks for making me read well. Thank you to my Tyndale family for allowing me to spread my wings and discover new territory. But most of all thank you for supporting my efforts.

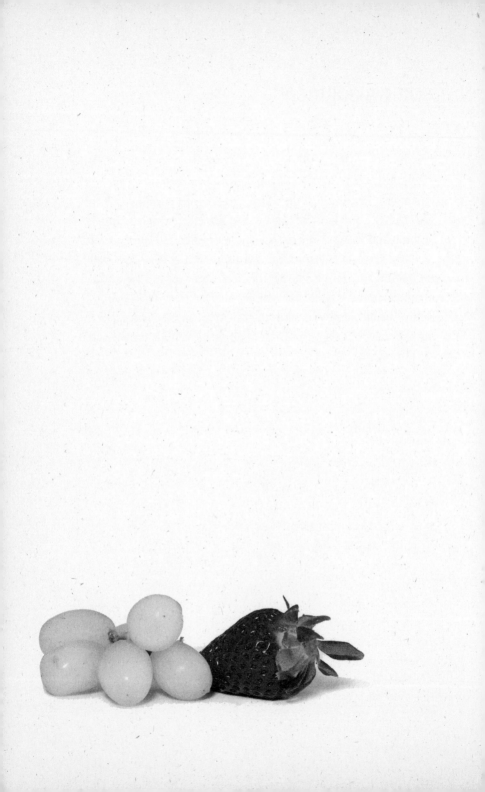

introduction

I believe there is a hormone specifically in women that scientists haven't discovered yet that has everything to do with our weight issues and our inability to resist temptation. I also believe that a crafty serpent in a lovely Garden long ago was smart enough to recognize this issue and capitalize on it. Small wonder that the first sin had to do with eating. Yup, from the time Eve took a chunk out of that piece of fruit (no one knows what it really was—apple, pear, grapes, figs, whatever the fruit), humans have struggled with what goes in and comes out of their mouths.[1]

Sigh! It is true I am a blatant offender; even as I watch my hips spread, I struggle with this thing inside of me crying out for more—more cream puffs, more cupcakes loaded with frosting, more of anything that will fight against my desire to be a perfect size eight.

Oh, rest assured, I've done the size-two thing and still wasn't satisfied. Nooo, I couldn't leave well enough alone. I had to *gain* weight. Twiggy hadn't made thin fashionable in my neighborhood when I was a teenager and in my early twenties. Back then, I wanted curves like my peers. So I ate. And ate. And ate. To no avail. I gained nothing. Nothing but a voracious appetite! And now, decades later when size two is only a memory, I am still battling that appetite I developed. (Oops, I just spilled ice cream on my keyboard.)

Anyway, as I was sharing, girlfriend, this whole diet thing is more than a notion. When my cute little svelte publisher approached me about doing a diet book, I didn't know if I should be offended or not. I mean, what was she trying to say? Was she suggesting I needed to lose weight or something? I talked the idea over with my mentor, who said, "You know, if you write that book, you're going to have to live it!" Aaargh! Would I be biting off more than I could really chew?

As you begin this book, I want to make sure you understand that I am not a nutritionist, okay? At the end of the list of all that I do—author, speaker, television cohost, relationship expert, empowerment coach, singer, blah, blah, blah—I am simply a woman who has called everyone from Jenny to Nutrisystem, joined the Weight Watchers of the world, been to South Beach and back. When it comes to diets, I've done them all. I've had successes and failures in various numbers and dress sizes. I, probably like you, have at least three sizes hanging in my closet for whichever direction I swing, but frankly I'm exhausted from the constant volleying—and I need more closet space.

So I decided to rise to the challenge to share with you what I've learned about the *D* word. Mm-hmm, it could be called the most maddening thing next to men—dieting. I'm going to share with you the real skinny on losing it, how to deal with whatever it may be that is keeping you away from the size you want to be, and how to win the battle with your hips and other body parts you don't like once and for all. Some of my observations may surprise you. This is more about getting to the heart of the matter than experimenting with temporary tricks. We are going to settle this weight thing for good. Tackle it to the floor and kill it. Free at last, free at last, yes, you are going to be free at last! Trust me—I'm going to push some buttons you may not want me to push. But if you'll be honest with me, I'll be honest with you, and we'll master this struggle together. Who knows, we may make it to the Oprah show (before she goes off the air) or one of those "new you" shows yet!

—*Michelle McKinney Hammond*

Looking in the Mirror

I WAS IN CRISIS, and I knew it. Pure envy and a smidge of hatred (did I say pure?) had filled my heart. There is nothing like being in a changing room filled with skinny little models to highlight your cellulite and take what your thighs really look like to a whole other level.

Here I was, modeling for a fund-raiser for my girlfriend, renowned designer Barbara Bates, and having a weight crisis before hitting the runway. I was one of the "celebrity models." Meanwhile, the real models, little waifs with absolutely no body fat, paraded around in their thong underwear with no bras, naked and unashamed, while I bolted to the darkest corner I could find to try on my ensemble. Yes, I admit it: I looked. I stared. I swallowed the lump in my throat and thought back to when I had been that size. Then I headed for the table laden with a spread of hors d'oeuvres and reached for something with cream in it. Hey, my motto is *If you can't join them, eat something.*

The words from one of the millions of diet books I'd read came back to me: *Observe how skinny people eat and imitate them.* Those skinny little nymphs never went near the table of hors d'oeuvres.

The one that finally sidled over to peruse the spread settled for one pitiful little grape. One grape! What was that supposed to do? One grape wouldn't know what to do in my system; it would have too much room to float around. It is a horrible thing to feel trapped in one's own body and not know how to get out. Watching what skinny people ate was not working for me; it only made me frustrated. And yes, observing thin people's eating habits made me eat more while my body image plummeted to even greater depths.

Oh, I knew how to dress up my weight issues. I cleaned up well, believe me. I knew every trick in the book, from my scientifically constructed undergarment foundation that had promised to take me down three dress sizes in three minutes (and did) to wearing the right colors and lines to appear smaller than I really was. Even as others looked me up and down, approvingly cooing, "Ooo, did you lose weight?" I knew the real deal. The minute I unsnapped that bad sister (my undergarment), the awful truth would once again explode. The truth of the matter was that I was naked and *very* ashamed. I was fat! Quiet as it was kept, after all the sucking it up and dressing it up, there was no way around what my mirror and I intimately knew.

Now most people would say, "Michelle, what is the big deal? You're not really fat. You are the average size of most of America! Men still think you are fine. When they stop looking, you're in trouble, but until then, get a grip, girl!" But in my mind I was fat, and that is all that mattered. Because I was used to being so much smaller, weight and size were all relative. You have to understand that I graduated from high school weighing 103 pounds. Did you hear what I just said? 103. That is one-zero-three. Many moons and many pounds later, I can tell you that 103 is a very vague memory. And though you live in the skin you're in, you never get used to the new you. Your mind keeps reminding you of "the way we were."

I could sympathize with Princess Diana, who went to extremes to lose weight after deciding she didn't like how she looked on camera. I could second that motion. Trust me, for every woman who has ever said to me, "Oh, you are so much prettier in person! Did you lose weight?" I cursed the camera that added ten pounds, and then I cursed myself for not getting rid of the ten pounds that would make me look on the screen the way I did in person.

Image is everything. It defines us and validates us, or so we think. It affects our self-esteem, our moods, the way we carry and present ourselves to others, and even the way we interact and love. It can make or break a relationship. It's true. I recall meeting this cute French man one Christmas holiday. He thought I was the most beautiful woman in the world until my own self-loathing drove me to show him photos of a much thinner me, just to prove I was really cute, in case he didn't think I was beautiful enough. His encouragement for me to diet didn't do a lot for the relationship, I can tell you that. Though I was the perpetrator of his desire to see a smaller version of me, I held it against him and no longer felt comfortable or beautiful. Did it make me stop eating? Absolutely not. I got rid of him and kept the food. It was more comforting. It loved me back . . . or did it?

As I stood in front of the mirror looking at my lushness in all its glory, berating and insulting myself, it was as if my supersonic spiritual hearing were open. I heard the voice of God. I am not lying to you. He said, "Michelle, if you were at an art museum looking at a painting and the artist were present, would you talk in negative terms about what he had created?"

"Of course not!" I answered.

"Why not?" He asked.

"Because I wouldn't want to hurt the artist's feelings?" I muttered.

"Well," He said. "I am the artist of you, and I'm standing here with you. I created you fearfully and wonderfully. You were good and perfect in My eyes until you got ahold of yourself. Don't insult My creation. The parts that you don't like are the works of your own hands, so do something about it." Talk about a slap in the face! He was right. I was the one who had added stuff to the canvas that He had not put there. It was not my body's fault it looked the way it did; it was my fault. I kept feeding it. It simply complied to all my offerings. There it was. The cold, hard facts. The ugly truth. Ah, but the truth can set you free if you let it.[1]

I don't know about you, but God talks to me a lot when I'm looking in the mirror, perhaps because that is where victory will always begin. One of my favorite songs by Michael Jackson says exactly that. I have to look at the woman in the mirror and decide to make the change. It begins with me. It begins with you. We're making a simple decision and remaining committed to our commitment. Sounds simple, but it's not that easy, and we all know it. A lot of things stand in the way of us and our commitment. Throughout this book, we'll take a look at those things one by one. But in the meantime, it's time to get real with yourself once and for all.

KEEPING IT REAL

- What do you think of yourself? How do you really feel about your present state of being?

- How does your physical image compare with the image you have of yourself in your head?

- How driven or motivated are you by other people's opinions of your image?

- What needs to happen to make you reconcile where you are to where you want to be?

- What is a realistic goal of what you would like to look like?

DIVA REFLECTIONS

My girlfriend Vanessa always says, "I'm not fat. I'm just fluffy." Sometimes when you're not happy with where you are, a little humor goes a long way until you get moving toward your goal.

The Real Issue

ONCE UPON A TIME there was a woman who had an issue. Girl, I'm not talking about you; I'm talking about another woman, okay? Anyway, she had had this issue for a long time. She had struggled and sought help from various sources to no avail; she only ended up worse for the wear, living in the isolation that comes from wearing out people with our issues. One day she heard that this man who healed people was coming to town, so she pressed her way through the crowd to grab hold of his garment. Well, instantly her issue was solved. She could feel it. She was healed! It was a miracle! But now she had a new problem. The man wanted to know who had been pulling on his clothing. Humbly, she stepped forward and told him "the whole truth."

Hmm, what truth did she tell? And why did she have to tell him all her business? She knew it was time to face her issue once and for all, call it what it was, and put it to rest. She knew that acknowledging what had led her to the state she was in was critical to maintaining her healing. Usually the *issue* is just the fruit that grows from the root of something we've ignored or overlooked.

There is always a story behind the issue. There was something to learn from this woman's issue. Can I get an amen?

You may have guessed by now that I'm referring to the biblical story about the woman with the issue of blood.[1] The stranger who healed her was Jesus. I've always been fascinated with this story, not just because I'm nosy and wanted to know what the real deal was with this woman, but because of the story surrounding this incident. The chapter actually starts with Jesus going to see a young girl who is at the point of dying. Keep in mind that this girl is *twelve years old*. On His way to see the young girl, the woman with the issue stops Him. The woman has been struggling with her issue for *twelve years*. Just as the woman is healed, Jesus receives news that the child has died. The news interrupts the conversation the newly healed and whole woman is having with Jesus. Jesus leaves the woman, goes and raises the child from the dead, and commands her parents to feed her.

I've read this story several times. The same thought always comes to mind. In some sort of spiritual way, I think the woman and the little girl are connected. Mm-hmm. There is something charming about the girlish nature of a woman until that little girl begins to act out. It can rob a woman of her victory. You see, childlike and childish are two different things. Yet for most of us there is some area of arrested development—something that makes us act childishly—that endangers our health, wealth, and wholeness and affects our quality of life based on the responses we have to the things life brings our way. The number twelve was the common denominator in both the woman's and the little girl's stories. This number is spiritually significant regarding government or a thing being established or becoming law (think twelve tribes of Israel and the twelve disciples—they were foundational in establishing God's Kingdom in the Old Testament and the New Testament). Past experiences or reoccurring disappointments can develop grounded beliefs that become "law" to us and drive our behavior. This childish behavior can keep us from gaining or keeping the victory we crave so deeply. Maturity demands that we make different choices, exercise different disciplines, and stop having knee-jerk reactions. As mature women, we have to deal with certain harsh realities and not allow the way we think and respond to be mastered by our emotions. It is not until we are willing to put to rest certain childish notions and habits and feed ourselves with a healthier mind-set that we can move on to the wholeness we all long for. This can be an ongoing issue for years or until you get tired of being sick and tired.

I remember the day many years ago when I sat in a counselor's chair at Diet Center, my latest endeavor to get rid of extra pounds. I was determined to get on top of my weight. I had finally concluded—after trying the gamut of fad diets that worked for a minute before heaping back on more pounds than I had lost—that I needed supervision. The slim lady sitting opposite me at the center was so nice. She leaned in, speaking in hushed tones, almost conspiratorially, as if this were our little secret and we were in this together. That was *soooo* not true. My arm couldn't fit into one of her pant legs! The more she went over the diet plan with me, the more I fought against the urge to weep. This sense of mourning that I couldn't explain just washed over me. It came from somewhere deep within as if I were saying farewell to a deeply loved friend, although I had never called the roll on my stomach that. I fought back the tears, afraid that if I let out one sigh, I would end up on the floor, bawling my eyes out.

"Anything else?" she smiled as she summed up her instructions and handed me my bags of prepackaged salad dressings, pills to boost my metabolism, and booklets of instructions and menus. I silently shook my head and rose from my chair, afraid that if I said anything, I would explode. "Well, you just call if you have any questions, and I'll see you next week." Again I wordlessly nodded, managed a weak smile, and fled before I burst into tears.

Leaning against the bathroom stall, I wondered what my meltdown was all about. I felt as if I were in a spiritual tug-of-war like the wicked witch in *The Wizard of Oz*, who screamed, "Help, I'm melting," when Dorothy splashed her with water. I think my fat was recoiling from the thought of finally meeting its demise. Something inside of me knew this was it. This was D-day. I was going to lose the weight, but then what?

Though I wanted to lose weight, I felt sad at the prospect. Why was this such a fight for me? Why was I suddenly consumed with fear and angst? That was when it struck me. My issue with food was more than pleasure seeking gone out of control. It was a safety issue. I felt safe when I was fat, even though I didn't like the way I looked. My fat kept me out of trouble. As a little underweight girl in school, I had been prey for bullies. I felt helpless because of my size. I didn't stand a chance against those who were significantly larger than me. I spent most of my childhood trying to put on weight to no avail. So I hid behind hefty friends, relying on them to keep me safe. They were more formidable foes to those who threatened me. I was the brunt of jokes. I was "Little Bit" and "Weasel." One day in art class, we took turns drawing one another; when my turn came to be the model, the guys snickered and drew straight lines while someone yelled, "We can't see her." It was a very traumatic time I wouldn't relive for millions of dollars. I was a foreigner with a heavy West Indian accent, too smart, bucktoothed, and too skinny. Not a pretty picture. And worse than the fear was the loneliness I felt in my isolated world of a place called "different." Little did I know, Little Bit wouldn't last for long. Age and hormonal changes made up for what my figure lacked as I turned the bend into womanhood and left childhood behind.

All of a sudden at the age of eighteen, I had curves! And those curves attracted all types of men I wasn't ready to deal with. I was used to being ignored. All of a sudden the tables had turned. I was overwhelmed by all the attention and naive about making the right choices. With each relationship disappointment, my weight began to increase. Before I realized it, by the time I reached twenty-two, I had the opposite weight problem, and the seesaw dieting began between relationships.

As an adult no longer afraid of bullies, another danger loomed nonetheless. Now my fat protected me from the wrong men and the drama that came with them. My realization after the visit to Diet Center was that a new, skinny me would once again be vulnerable to those men and wrong decisions that seemed bigger than my capacity to overcome or even resist. If I could subconsciously disqualify myself from the attention of those things that got me into trouble, I wouldn't have to deal with them.

There, I've said everything out loud, "the whole truth," or at least I've made a good start. As often as I had joked about the fact that, if you had to be in an awful relationship, you should at least be able to enjoy the view, no gorgeous man is really worth your health's being in jeopardy. Why should he walk away from the relationship looking as fine as when he entered and leave you looking worse for the wear? And no temptation or person should have the power to drive you toward an unhealthy lifestyle—such as being overweight. You're going to have to weather the tests in your life one way or another without succumbing to self-degradation. Think about it. Anyway, that's a sampling of my truth, my issue. What about you? What is really at the core of your weight issue?

It's easy enough to blame it on your mother's insisting you clean your plate or your respect for people starving in Ethiopia. Of course, there is truth to a woman's body changing at different stages of her life, so you can blame it on menopause, men on pause, or whatever. There are a multitude of excuses one could hide behind. But the truth of the matter is that, at the end of the day, the reason you are not at your desired weight lurks deep within you—not in the pit of your stomach but in your subconscious. The truth lies in an experience or experiences that trigger you to abuse your body by overeating, not eating enough, or just having enough bad eating habits to make your metabolism pack up all its toys and abdicate its post. There is a reason your body is not cooperating with you, and we are going to get down to the real nitty-gritty together.

I say, no matter how ugly or ridiculous your issue sounds, let it out and let the healing begin!

KEEPING IT REAL

Think back to when weight first became an issue for you.

- What event triggered a change in how you ate? How did you feel at the time?

- When did you notice the change in your body?

- What was your reaction? the reaction of others? How did it make you feel about yourself?

- Is food a comfort or a punishment for you? Why? What triggers your bad eating habits?

- Where can you redirect your focus when you feel like eating the wrong things?

DIVA REFLECTIONS

Learn to accept your humanity without making excuses for it. Every broken place in our lives has the potential to be even stronger once it mends. Take advantage of your brokenness, and exploit it to the fullest measure. Remember, for every sad story you have, someone has a sadder one. Share yours, free yourself, and the pounds will flee.

3

Naked and Ashamed

ONE OF THE MOST troublesome deceptions in life is that "the grass is always greener on the other side." Who came up with that idea, anyway? And why didn't anyone take a walk over to the other side to find out if it was true and what made the grass greener if that was indeed fact? And really, is it *always* greener? That's pretty hard to believe. Perspective is everything.

In hindsight, I won't say how many pounds later, I was pretty okay skinny. That's right. I looked fine when I was in school. I think most of those folks messing with me were "haters." Mm-hmm, they were just mad 'cause they couldn't squeeze into the cute little things I got to wear because of my petite state. The guys just didn't get me because they were surrounded by amazons, so that was their norm. Yes, the lightbulb went on as I sat looking through a school yearbook one day. I realized I was actually pretty cute back then. I didn't know what all my angst had been about.

The deeper truth is that I responded more to external pressure than to internal peace. I allowed the opinions of others to shape how I saw myself. And that is when the trouble began. Now when I see models that look like I did back in the day, I think to myself,

Was I crazy or what? I could have been a model like them and made some money! And why did a few pounds matter so much? Here's proof that we are never satisfied. Once I started gaining weight, I panicked to the other extreme. At a size eight, I was still small (and probably the perfect size) in the eyes of some people, but because everything is relative to where you've been, I felt gargantuan. And so the weight fluctuations began every time I felt the squeeze from my favorite outfits. If I had never started dieting, I would not have ended up on this roller coaster in the first place. I killed my metabolism early for nothing. Why was I on a diet when I was wearing a size eight? Somebody tell me!

It's an age-old dilemma. I think, again, it started back in that doggone garden.[1] That garden was paradise until that old, slimy snake showed up making all his suggestions that led to that fatal snack that made Adam and Eve look at each other funny. Think about it. They had been prancing around in that garden in front of each other naked for God knows how long. After a couple of bites of a piece of fruit, they ran for cover and became embarrassed by their nakedness. When they apologized to God for their nakedness, God simply asked, "Who told you that you were naked?" Oooh! That's right! Who told you there was something wrong with you? Was it your mama? a peer? or you? And who determines what is true and right? Obviously Adam and Eve were really naked, so I think God was really asking them, "What's wrong with you being naked? And why isn't it all right with you?" Good question. Being naked hadn't bothered them before. Why did it bother them now? What had made the difference?

Could it be the big *C* word? That's right—comparison. See, the snake got Eve to compare herself to God. That is what got her in trouble—comparing herself to something (or Someone) that was so beyond her. Something she couldn't do anything about. Something that really didn't amount to a hill of beans in the grand scheme of things. I mean, if she could be like God, would that have made her God? Absolutely not! She would have been even more disgruntled to discover that, even though she was *like* Him, she still had to be *subject* to Him. As they say, you should always be careful what you ask for or wish for or desire to be like. There is always a curse along with the blessing. To whom much is given, much is required.[2] But back to the story and the point.

Comparison is false shame. It gathers shame from a place that has no basis for it. Comparing ourselves always leads to dissatisfaction. Dissatisfaction is the slippery slope that always leads to our demise. It colors our attitudes and affects our choices in detrimental ways. We take strange measures to live up to standards that exist only inside of our own heads. C'mon, do blondes really have more fun? Ask Elizabeth Taylor or Sandra Bullock or several other raven-haired or copper-tressed women.

I have a girlfriend named Kim who was the first large-size model for Ebony Fashion Fair, one of the world's largest traveling fashion shows. Kim is a big sister—a big, gorgeous, sexy sister. Men fall all over themselves, running behind her like schoolboys. Kim is one of the most confident women I know. She wears formfitting clothes and flaunts every curve she has, while I schlep behind her shrouded in layers. The same thing happens with my travel assistant Jennifer, a big, beautiful girl. She is cool and confident, always dressed to the nines with accessories to match. The girl is hot, okay?! When Jennifer and I walk through the airport, guys lose their balance because they are checking out this chick. As a matter of fact, once we got separated on a trip, and she met this fine-looking brother in the airport while she was waiting for the next flight . . . the rest is history! Meanwhile, I'm still trying to make peace with my body image and keeping all my stuff under wraps. (Okay, I see you all signing up to travel with me now. . . .)

All of that to say, beauty is as beauty does. If beauty waited to be praised, it would wither under the glare of many who didn't recognize it. Ah, but when beauty owns its own wonderfulness, everyone celebrates it. Again, perception is everything. It's called value perception in advertising. If you price something too cheaply, no one wants it because they don't believe it is worth anything. Even if it were worth a lot, the low price creates suspicion that it is not authentic. Now price a piece of junk at a ridiculously high price, and watch people scramble to have it. Uh-huh, the same is true of how you view and carry yourself. On a day when I don't feel beautiful, I am invisible. No one says anything to me. But on a day that I feel good about myself, I may not even really look my best, but all of a sudden I'm getting compliments right and left! Go figure.

This is not something we spend a lot of time thinking about, but it is imbedded in us; from the time we are little girls playing with our first Barbie dolls, the pressure to look a certain way begins. The model for what is beautiful is established in our minds as we style Barbie's hair, preparing her for her first date with flawless Ken. The figures 36-24-36 are the standard, do or die. And while parts of that figure can now be purchased, we are never good enough. Beautiful enough. Desirable enough. Slim enough . . . Enough already!

In my opinion, the pressure to look a certain way has gotten even worse in the present day, leading many a starlet to throw up perfectly good food in order to stay painfully thin. I'm telling you now, the peach cobbler is staying down in my stomach where I put it! Looking good should never put your health in danger or make you lose your dessert. It's time to uncover the lies that have taken root in your psyche and are leading you down irrational paths of yo-yo dieting. Just remember that whenever the yo-yo dips, it bounces up higher than where it was originally, and so does our weight. So let's take a deep breath and repeat after Popeye, "I yam what I yam!" That's a good place to start. No looking to the left or the right. Let's take an objective look at ourselves. Let's remove all other pictures from our minds and decide what we are going to do about *us*. After all, the only person you can control is yourself—and that is work enough.

KEEPING IT REAL

- When did you first compare yourself to someone else? What was it about that person that you admired?

- What attributes do you possess that others celebrate? Are you able to celebrate them too?

- How does comparison affect your self-esteem? Are your comparisons realistic? Would it be possible for you to achieve what you envy?

- Without comparisons, what does your ideal self look like?

- What would you have to do to achieve your goal? How badly do you want to? How will you begin?

DIVA REFLECTIONS

Remember this—there will always be someone smaller than you, bigger than you, wider than you, shorter, taller, cuter, smarter, wittier, richer—you name it—more than you. This leads to the very first *maaaaajor* thing you must do for yourself. Walk up to the mirror, and take a good look at your reflection. Accept what you see standing there. You may or may not ever change, so determine to be the best you that you can be in your present state. Kill the green-eyed monster, and remind yourself that no one can do *you* better than you, no matter what size they are, and get on with the business of living without comparison.

4

A Shadow of My Former Self

ALL RIGHT, I am going to follow my own advice. I am going to take stock of all the things that I could celebrate about myself right here and now. I've accomplished a lot. I am not the woman I once knew. I am a lot wiser than before. I am indeed a shadow of my former self, although my "self" is casting a larger shadow than before. I've written more than thirty-five books, cohosted an Emmy Award–winning talk show for ten years, won numerous awards in the advertising world for radio and television commercials I created back in the day, am currently respected as a life and relationship empowerment coach . . . the list goes on, but I am reduced to a state of being "verklempt," or should I say horrifyingly perplexed, about my weight. I mean, I have solved the problems of countless men and women, and I have a few suggestions for the world, but pardon the pun, it seems I've bitten off more than I can chew when it comes to mastering my weight. And I am not alone. No, no, no. How is it that women can become Supreme Court justices, walk on the moon, and birth babies (which is the most complex achievement of all) and still not be able to get on top of their issues with weight? What is that all about?

Some will blame having children for their lack of ability to bounce back to their former selves, but famous *Project Runway* model superstar Heidi Klum puts that argument to rest. Didn't you just want to slap her when she modeled for Victoria's Secret eight weeks after she'd had a baby? (Forgive me, Jesus, but the green monster escaped from his hiding place for a minute.) But seriously, everybody was talking about how quickly Heidi's body snapped back, which only deepened my comparison issues. However, every time she says, "One day you're in, the next you're out," and kisses another fledgling designer on her show good-bye ever so graciously, I forgive her and love her all over again. "Well," you might say in her defense (or yours), "that Heidi was only thirty-two years old, and she had enough money to pay people to help her snap her body back." True dat. But there are ordinary people doing the same thing without the help of chefs and trainers or supposedly supernatural genes. What's their secret?

I don't know about you, but I've evolved on several levels—emotionally, spiritually, professionally, and financially. But physically? I remain stuck at ground zero looking in my closet at my favorite suit that I haven't been able to wear for two years—but I'm keeping hope alive! Barbra Streisand sang it best, "Can it be that it was all so simple then . . . or has time rewritten every line?" Somewhere along the way between the thirty and forty marker, I had lost control of my weight and didn't even realize it. The saying goes that those who forget their past are destined to repeat it. So let's start at the beginning and retrace our steps to see just where we lost that control.

There was a time in my life when I ate to live, not lived to eat. When I was in high school and college, I had no money, so my social life had to revolve around something other than eating. Ahhh, I just heard a collective sigh rise in the room. How much of our lives now revolves around eating? *Let's do lunch! How about dinner?* It is amazing how much food we put away in the name of having a social life. When I was in school, my social life revolved around activities—going to football and basketball games where I burned a ton of calories screaming my head off for my favorite team. I was a pom-pom girl, and I played and marched in the high school band. I went to every dance and party whether I was invited or not. (And let me tell you, I went to dance, not social- ize!) I was on the track team, in the school play, and in every talent show. . . . Whew! I'm exhausted just thinking about all the activities. I ate less and was more active. No wonder I was thin. I was always idling on high. Eating was something my parents forced me to do, otherwise I forgot. Unlike my peers, I didn't like sweets. My perfect idea of a snack was a glass of milk and a hand- ful of lettuce before bed. Yes, even my mother said I was weird. I didn't like a lot of things, so that narrowed my options of what I ate when I finally did.

Aha! That was it! Back in the day, I ate to live. I did not live to eat. Don't hate me 'cause I'm telling the truth. Trust me. That way of eating had long fallen by the wayside to be replaced by some things that would not contribute to my girlish figure of yonder years. As I got older—and less active—I still didn't really care for sweets, but the few I indulged in were loaded with fat. Some of them included ice cream, cheesecake, crème caramel or flan, cup- cakes from my fave local spots (ooh, just the thought of them sets me off!), caramel sundaes from Mickey D's, chocolate-dipped cones from Dairy Queen, an occasional Kit Kat whenever I was feeling hormonal. I hope I'm not being a bad influence. This is supposed to be a diet book, and you know what talking about food does to us. Suffice it to say, you get the picture. Though I thought I was indulging in a cultured selection of fare, it was nevertheless deadly to a girl in search of a small waistline and low cholesterol. Add to this list anything with a rich sauce or lots of cheese and my ultimate Achilles' heel—bread laden with butter. . . . Well, small wonder, which I was not, I looked the way I did.

This trip down memory lane and my past habits all came to me as I looked at an old photo in my album. When I was active and young, I had a firm jawline. I had Michelle Obama arms and flaunted them shamelessly in a halter. What happened?

"Lord, I want those arms back," I sighed. That's when I heard Him. Yes, that would be God. He was talking to me again.

"If you give me your body for forty days, I will give them back to you."

"Exactly what does that mean, Jesus. What would that look like?" I queried.

"I want to cleanse your palate," He said. I agreed with Him that my palate was pretty corrupted.

I heard Him say, "For the next forty days you are to eat only fruit and vegetables and drink only water."

"That's it?" I gasped.

"Yup, that's it!" (Now just in case you don't believe God says "yup," I can tell you He does when He's talking to me—have your own conversation!)

He continued: "Michelle, that means no cream, no potatoes, rice, bread, sugar; all the stuff that's smothered your food and slain your palate is not allowed. Not only will this be good for you physically, it will be great for you spiritually." Well! That was the end of the discussion.

So, I read the story about Daniel in the Bible; he had done the same diet when he went down to Babylon to be a slave.[1] He decided to refuse all the rich food that was being sent to him from the king's table and chose simpler fare—namely, vegetables and water. He wagered with the eunuchs watching him that he would be in better condition than his fellow prisoners after ten days. After ten days, Daniel and the three friends that had joined him on the diet looked healthier and better nourished than the other guys who had been eating everything they had been given. Daniel and his friends were also mentally sharper—go figure! They didn't have a lot of rich and heavy food clouding their thoughts. I so related to those guys.

That became my story—veggies, fruit, and water. The pounds fell off! I didn't even have to exercise. I chose to eat raw, so I just chowed down on great salads and fruit mixtures, being careful to eat more vegetables than fruit. I put fruit in the water to flavor it and drank chamomile tea without sugar when I needed to feel as if I were really drinking something yummy. My taste buds sharpened; it was as if I tasted everything on a whole other level. After the first week, I didn't miss sweets. My energy level shot through the ceiling. I was getting on my own nerves. No longer lethargic, I had strength to spare. My mind sharpened, and I actually remembered things! (Some of you will get that now, and some of you will understand that much later in life.)

During my time of eating only veggies and fruit, my skin got clear, my eyes were shining, and I was looking too cute for myself! Everyone was exclaiming over my new fashion-plate look. I came out of hiding behind my layers and put on formfitting clothes to show off. I felt fabulous and looked even better. I had cheekbones! And arms I could show! My waist reappeared! "Ooo, what did you do?" people cooed. I shared with them what I had done—a short litany—fruit, vegetables, and water. Their faces went blank. "That's it? What else did you eat?"

"That's it," I said.

"Well, you look wonderful," they said, backing away as if to ward off any suggestions that they do the same.

They had no need to worry; I understood that my dietary restrictions were my light to walk in and not to be forced on others. I finished my commitment to eat as God had instructed me for forty days with flying colors. My self-esteem was through the ceiling. Shoot, I was fine! You couldn't tell me nothin'.

I had some ice cream to celebrate . . . and then one thing led to another and . . .

Uh-huh, you know where I'm going already, don't you? All the diets will work, but if nothing in you dies while you are dieting, your fat will be back to haunt you. It's just like a bad horror movie when the woman who's been chased finally thinks her tormentor is dead and she leans forward to take one last look . . . wham! His hand reaches up and grabs her. Yes, I was screaming six months after my fruit-and-veggie fast when my new, slim clothing had grown too tight and all I had left was a memory of my former self. I had missed the point of the entire exercise. That's when I learned that it's one thing to cleanse your palate, but it's quite another to keep it clean. However, where there is a will, there is a way—we just have to get a few things out of the way in order to find the path to getting it off and keeping it off.

KEEPING IT REAL

- What does your "shadow" (as in your favorite size) look like? What did you do then that you don't do now?

- How badly do you want to reclaim your former self? What would you need to do to get back to that image or a happy medium?

- Make a list of your favorite foods. Separate the junk from the good stuff. Be honest with yourself about the balance of what you eat— more junk or nutritious food?

- Review how you used to eat when you liked your size. Assess how your eating habits have changed as your body has changed and what you need to adjust.

- Try my purge or another method of doing a cleanse. There are lots of great herbal kits on the market at your health stores. Note how you feel while you're doing it. (Depending on how toxic your system has become, you might feel worse before you feel better, but persevere!) Never attempt any of this without consulting your doctor.

- Make a list of activities you can enjoy with friends that do not include eating.

DIVA REFLECTIONS

I don't know about you, but in some ways I think I look a whole lot better now, even though I was smaller before. Somewhere in the middle of life there's this wonderful place called finding a happy medium. But even greater yet is finding a better you—a new you. Why reinvent the old wheel when you can have a new and better model? One that makes wiser choices that make you feel better physically and emotionally. So pick your battles with yourself, come to a realistic conclusion, and then go for it! Remember a healthier body is a great gift to give to yourself, not just because you should, but simply because you can. Close your eyes and say it to yourself. *Yes, we can!*

5

Putting Away Childish Things

IT'S TRUE: Bad habits die hard. How could I get back to cute only to find myself ascending up the scale, seemingly by leaps and bounds, once again? You would think after I noticed I had gained five pounds that I would have put myself back on lockdown and stopped the avalanche right then and there, but nooooo . . . twenty pounds later. . . . This is why I think we love Oprah so much. We have swung the weight pendulum with her. She is one of us. My girl has fought the fight and gone splat with the rest of the women of the world who battle the same weight issues. Depending on our heart condition, we've envied her, perhaps even been a "hater" after she dropped major pounds, and comforted ourselves by thinking, *She'll be back.* Like hawks we circled our televisions, watching and waiting for the first hint of an extra pound. When it happened, we said, "Could it be? Has sister girl put on a few pounds?" Once we concluded that indeed she had, we breathed a little easier, feeling at one with her again. It was official; we now had permission to be average-size women.

And though the war rages with Oprah, you, and me, the greater question is, how can we all stop the pendulum from swinging?

And why does it swing at all? I just said it. We are in a war. Get your boat off that river of Denial and find a new stream called Reality, girl! It's not just about you eating too much, or liking bread and potatoes more than you should; this is war! It's a war between your inner child and the woman you've become. It's a war between your flesh and your spirit. You've heard the saying the spirit is willing but the flesh is weak.[1] The devil may want you fat, but God does not. When you scratch beneath the surface, you will discover that losing weight is going to take more than a made-up mind. It is going to take a submitted spirit, too. And your mind and spirit have to line up with your will to exercise another *D* word we hate. I can't even type it, but I must . . . d-d-d-d-discipline. Whew! My fingers are still aching. Just typing the word made me hungry!

Case in point: I have three dogs—Milan, my baby girl, and Matisse and Micah, my little boys. Now Matisse and Micah are lean and mean. They don't have any issues with weight. Don't you just hate men for that? I think beer bellies are a woman's ultimate revenge—a one-two punch. (Take that for being thin naturally; take that for pregnancy.) Yes, beer bellies can be a beautiful thing to even out the score. Anyway, as I was saying, my boys have no problems with weight. Milan, however, is just like her mom (that would be me). She's short and stacked with junk in her trunk. (That would be a little extra padding in the caboose area.) When the veterinarian told me she needed to lose two pounds, I was mortified. I had been telling her she wasn't fat, just fluffy—to her detriment.

The problem came when I tried to get a handle on Milan's diet by cutting back her portions. It didn't work. I couldn't figure out why. Then I sat and watched all the dogs eating their dinner one day. Milan finished what was in her bowl, then she continued grazing from Micah's and Matisse's bowls. All three of them wandered from bowl to bowl, which made it hard to keep track of who was eating how much, but in the end I realized that Milan was eating more than everybody else. No wonder she was gaining instead of losing! I realized I had to retrain them to stick to eating from their own bowls. This became a major project. They rebelled. I wondered if their food tasted better to them when they were pilfering from one another's bowls. It just wasn't fun to stick to one bowl, it seemed. Milan became so upset every time I gently guided her back to her own bowl that she went on a hunger strike. The boys were bewildered as well but ended up being quite happy with the arrangement and seemed to revel in putting their heads down in their bowls and not coming up until they were finished. There was something to be said for eating uninterrupted, it seemed. They then reverently checked one another's bowls to see if there was anything left. Upon finding nothing, Matisse burped a satisfied burp and went in search of water. Meanwhile Milan had dug in her heels, refusing to eat. So I put her unfinished bowl away until the next mealtime. Did I say I had no children? I lied.

This exercise was repeated several times before Milan came to the conclusion that I was really serious. Once she figured out who was the boss, she lined up and began to submit to the new arrangement.

Your stomach is like Milan, Matisse, and Micah. It wants what it wants and will fight you for it. It is like a child. You know the kind. You've seen them in the grocery store, embarrassing their mothers—screaming, falling all out on the floor as if somebody were trying to kill them. Your heart is like that—incorrigible and insistent, influencing your mind and your stomach that you've got to have another bite and another and another and then thanking you with heartburn, acid reflux, and a bloated midsection. You have got to take control!

Let's start with the mind, because it is the commander. The

heart is out of control; therefore, you need to take a stand. Your emotions are supposed to follow the decisions made by your mind, not the other way around. But most of the time, what do we do? That's right—we follow our emotions, which will always get us in trouble. If you succumb to this, I have to tell you like it is—you are being a big baby. Babies get hungry. They cry. Babies get wet. They cry. They do not tolerate discomfort or inconvenience. Every need they have is urgent as far as they know, and they demand immediate attention and consolation. They haven't learned yet that being wet or hungry for a few minutes is not going to kill them. Neither will it kill us. And yet we act as if we don't know that. How many times have you said, "I'm starving!" and gone in search of anything—and I mean anything—to eat? Let's get real. We don't know what starving is. That is an insult to people who really are starving. Couple that with the fact that we just want what we want, even if it is killing us (literally), and we'll conclude that we sound ridiculous when we claim we are starving.

Remember the story I told you about Jesus and the little girl in Mark 5? After He raised her from the dead, He instructed her parents to feed her. Again, it's not about killing the child; it's about reeducating the child. It's also about reeducating your heart, your mind, and your palate. One of my friends has a husband who is overweight. This bothers him so much that he refuses to go out in public with her because he is ashamed of how he looks. This is sad because he is a nice-looking man who imagines himself to look like something other than what we see. I told him I had embarked on an eating plan with a company called Seattle Sutton. They prepare fresh meals within the calorie count that you want and deliver them fresh to your home every week. I was sharing with him how delicious I found the meals to be and that the bigger plus was that I was losing weight. He decided to try them out. Three days later he wrote me, saying, "Wow, Michelle, I thought you said the food was good. I forgot to tell you I've been living off of two quarts of Pepsi a day, soul food, and sweets. I haven't had a salad since 1932!" I wrote him back and said, "I suppose you should pronounce your taste buds dead! You are going to have to reeducate your palate to like things that are good for you." I suggested he go on a cleanse first so that his taste buds could be revived to appreciate the taste of fresh vegetables and cleaner food. I was informed a week later that he had abdicated the entire thing and gone back to his former regime. It didn't matter that he had lost four pounds in three days with Seattle Sutton. He just liked what he liked.

The apostle Paul in the Bible said something very profound one day when he was writing to one of the churches that he felt was careening out of control and not walking in love. He said, "When I was a child, I talked like a child, I thought like a child, I reasoned like a child. When I became a man, I put childish ways behind me."[2] What are some childish thoughts? I can think of several. How about these? I want it, therefore I should have it; I should have whatever I want and escape the consequences; I don't care how my wants impact anyone else. Yes, at the heart of a child is severe selfishness. Selfishness does not operate in love. It hurts even its loved ones because it is ruled by what it wants. That would be you I'm talking about. If you really loved yourself, you would stop hurting yourself.

This is what we couldn't understand as children when our parents punished or spanked us. They would say, "This is going to hurt me more than it's going to hurt you." Yeah, right. But it was true. Discipline was not fun for them, but they knew it was necessary because they had an idea of what they wanted us to look like as we grew up. It hurt me not to indulge my dog Milan when I knew that what would make her happy would also eventually make her sick. It hurt me not to give in to her, but I had a slimmer Milan in view who would look better and feel better. She couldn't see that far ahead. She lived in the immediacy of her desire. She was the child. I was the adult. I had to be responsible for her because she couldn't be responsible for herself.

One of the hardest things for us to grasp when it comes to this whole weight thing is lining up with the discipline it now demands for us to get the body we want. For most of us there was a day and time when we could eat whatever we felt like eating and nothing would happen. Now, however, you might as well just rub it right on your hips before putting it in your mouth, because that's where it's going to end up the minute it hits your intestinal tract. Yes, it's true, and I know it hurts, but take it for what it's worth. You can't do what you did before. Before, the way you ate was indulgence, but now it is abuse. You may not be walking around with bruises, but you are walking around with excess weight, which is really hurting you.

Sorry for stepping on your toes, but it is time to deal with the child in you. Sit her down, and talk to her gently. Let her know how much you love her. This is going to be hard for some of you. But you will never take good care of yourself until you love yourself enough to care about embracing the discipline it takes to get the results you want.

Every child I know responds to love the same way. The harder you are on them, the more they dig in their heels and resist correction. This is also true of adults. In the face of correction, we don't receive instruction well. We are too busy defending ourselves from feeling like failures. With this in mind, let's put a new spin on this whole weight-loss thing. While we are accepting the truth that some things must change externally, we are going to do some inner work first. We are going to choose to love ourselves just the way we are. We are going to stop being critical and mean to ourselves. We are going to stop seeing denial and discipline as punishment and embrace the *D* words as loving friends who are looking out for us. It all begins in our minds. Attitude is everything. Remember, you are no longer a child. You are a woman—a strong, confident woman who is in charge of her life and her inner child, and that inner child will only be released to charm people. In light of this new outlook, *no* is no longer a dirty word. It is an empowering declaration that proclaims, "We are the masters of our stomachs as well as our destinies." Denial is not a prison; it is actually liberating. Discipline is not an enemy but a friend who will escort us to where we really want to live—in a land called Healthy and Whole. And that, my friend, is not a fairy tale. That is real life—the good life.

KEEPING IT REAL

- Okay, check yourself. On a scale of one to ten, how disciplined are you about eating? How often do you eat three meals a day? How often do you stop eating when you are satisfied? How much of what you eat is healthy versus junk food? How much do you graze?

- How do you feel about discipline? What makes you rebel against it? How do you rationalize eating what you eat?

- What has been your attitude toward your body? Are you critical or loving? In what ways? What is the end result of your attitude toward yourself?

- What childish attitudes do you need to get rid of concerning your diet? What is a more realistic approach for you? What small steps can you begin to take so that you don't get overwhelmed?

- Write a promise to yourself to be kinder and gentler to yourself while moving toward your goal.

DIVA REFLECTIONS

It's amazing how our tastes can change. Once upon a time I thought sushi was the most disgusting food on the face of the earth. But my boyfriend liked it. So I learned to like it. Boyfriend's gone now, but I still crave sushi. It is definitely an acquired taste. The moral of this story? We can learn to love things that are good for us. As a child, I hated broccoli; now I love it. The bottom line is that our bodies will line up with what we decide to feed them. My dog whisperer, Erdem, always reminds me that I am the alpha or master of my dogs. Whenever I fail to act as if I'm the calm, confident leader in charge, my dogs run amuck and don't listen to me. But when I quietly take control, they sense I mean business and line up. Decide you mean business with your body. Remember that you are the boss.

The Heart of the Matter

I'M TAKING MY TIME walking through this whole heart, mind, spirit thing with you because, believe it or not, getting a healthy handle on these areas is the biggest part of gaining victory over your body. Have you ever fallen in love with something in the store, gotten it home, and wondered, *What was I thinking?* Mm-hmm, we've all done it. It was a moment when your heart deceived you into purchasing something you neither needed nor really wanted. The same thing happens when we go out to eat and our eyes become bigger than our stomachs. We end up ordering food we know we cannot finish, but at the time of ordering, we felt an urgency to have it. Your heart will lead you astray. It will deceive you and influence you to make decisions that are not in your best interest.

On one hand the heart is a slave driver; on the other it is a wimp, rolling over when you take charge of it. It's quite malleable and responds to established habits and ways of thinking. It literally will embrace whatever you decide if you choose to follow that course for any amount of time. People say it takes twenty-one days to form a habit, but real habits are cemented in the heart, not the intellect. The initial decision may be a mental one, but as the heart is made to consistently submit to your decision, at some point it will embrace your decision as a desire and natural inclination. It is consistency that makes things become a part of you. Think back to when you were little and your mother said, "You can't get up until you finish everything on your plate!" You lived under those directives for years. You finished what was on your plate whether you felt like it or not. Face it—some of us are still programmed to believe that. Whenever you feel full, something compels you to finish what's on your plate.

This did not become fully apparent to me until I did a diet program called Weigh Down. Some of the highlights of the program seemed simple enough until I had to exercise them. The first thing the program's guidelines said was that you should not eat until you are hungry. What?! What about the required three meals and two snacks a day that the other diet people rant and rave about? I'll answer that. They are actually right, and if you ate properly in the right portions, you would actually get hungry at the appropriate times. I discovered that my palate was not the only thing that was dead in my system. My stomach's alarm was broken too. Or perhaps *confused* was a better word. I either forgot to eat or waited until I was too hungry and then ate too much of all the wrong things. My stomach didn't know when it was hungry anymore; it was just grateful for whatever it got.

How do you know when you are really hungry? Details, details . . . I vaguely remember something about how the acids collect in your stomach when it's empty and cause it to growl. That's it. You are officially hungry when your stomach lets you know it is empty by growling. I couldn't remember the last time my stomach had growled. So I waited and waited and then voilà! It growled. I was so happy. I now had permission to eat. The next thing the program said was that you were not supposed to eat until you were stuffed;

you were supposed to eat until you were satisfied. Now I don't know about you, but I am a bit of an extremist. If I really, really like something, one is not enough. As with anything—from a potato chip to a shirt—if I like it, I indulge myself until the bag is empty, or I buy the same top in three different colors. So, not eating until I was stuffed was a totally different concept for me. But here is where my heart and lips came into play and ganged up on me.

My heart and lips said, *Hey if you like it, shovel it in. Let your taste buds dance until they can dance no more.* I was inclined to go along with this train of thought as long as the flavors on my tongue continued to abound. Now Weigh Down said that the stomach will actually tell you when there is enough food in it by sending a signal to your taste buds that actually affects the flavor of your food. Yes, that's right. It stops having the intensity of flavor and doesn't taste as good as it originally did because your stomach is too full to appreciate it. The problem was that I wasn't listening to my taste buds. I was listening to my heart. So I kept eating and eating until I felt I was about to burst at the gills.

I hated the uncomfortable feeling, but my heart was happy. This is how I broke the alarm in my stomach. It was so packed that it was having trouble processing everything I had stuffed into it. It only had so much acid allotted to break down the food I had practically inhaled and was at a loss as to what to do with the rest of the fare that settled there. Ah yes, that would be how the unprocessed food in my stomach just got stored as fat . . . hmmm. . . . Is anybody out there feeling me? Think about an overpacked washing machine. There's just not enough room for the water to move freely and clean every garment. This is why we do our laundry in loads. Well, the same thing applies to eating, but your heart will fool you into eating as if you will never see food again!

With these revelations in mind, I decided to go along with Weigh Down and see if what the program was saying held any import. Sure enough, I found some other good nuggets of truth from the program too. One nugget was that another way to help yourself was to eat your favorite stuff first so you wouldn't feel as if you had missed out on something when it was time to stop. Another thing the program suggested was that you put your utensils down between bites, chew slowly, and really savor the flavor of your food. Chew, chew, chew . . . No more shoveling it in. Perhaps part of the problem is that when we shovel down our food, we aren't really taking the time to experience the full flavor of every bite, so we get tricked into thinking we want to taste more.

Okay, so chew, chew, chew and savor the flavor. If you take the time to eat more slowly, the stomach can then process food as you send it down and get a better handle on when it has enough; then your stomach will let you know when enough is enough. However, when you eat quickly, the stomach can't figure it out fast enough to let you know in time. So there is a delay in the messaging, and this is why you go from enjoying your food to "Whew! I feel like a stuffed turkey. Just baste me and bake me!" Ever notice that many skinny people eat slowly and always get full fast? It's disgusting, isn't it? At first I used to feel guilty when I continued eating after skinny dinnermates pushed their plates back, but I quickly got over it. Oh, but that was the old me.

So what are we going to do now that we are allowing our minds to be renewed and educated? We are going to eat more slowly, master our hearts, and listen to our taste buds and our stomachs. We are going ask for doggy bags if we are in a restaurant and look forward to tasty leftovers the next time we get hungry or invest in some nice, inexpensive Glad storage bowls to stash away leftovers if we are at home. That way, when the heart starts whining about never seeing that tasty meal again, you can hold up the evidence in your hot little hands and say, "Oh, yes we will." Remember, grasshopper, you are the master of your heart. Not the other way around. It has to line up with your decisions. There is no such thing as the devil made you do anything. You just became a volunteer versus a victim of your own lusts, whichever way you want to put it; that's the gospel truth. The devil may wave it under your nose, but your hands grab the temptation.

Although what Weigh Down had to say made sense, it all sounded too simple. Something inside of me was trying to convince me that losing weight should be like a bad religious experience—self-flagellation and all. You know how some religious people can be. They are downright evil because they are not having any fun. They are too busy beating themselves up to have a joyous relationship with God and others. This mind-set translated over to dieting for me. I was convinced that I should feel like I suffered for every pound I lost, that I had paid a high, sacrificial price for each and every pound I shed. This was nothing more than pride. Pride insisted that I go through major gyrations so I could brag about what a great job I had done after I got the weight off. After all, what was the point if I couldn't win friends and influence people at the end of the day? Every magazine makes such a big deal over how so-and-so lost all her weight; my pride wanted me to be included in the numbers with the Kirstie Alleys and Valerie Bertinellis of the world—whether I had called Jenny or not. (That's another story for later.)

My pride issues had to be laid to rest before I listened to this advice. At this point I was desperate, and there's nothing like a little desperation to make you try something new. So I took a deep breath and let go of all my false religious notions, and I complied with the Weigh Down philosophy. I have to admit that, when I followed the simple guidelines, I lost weight. A lot of it! Go figure. I was doing so well that I began sharing Weigh Down's philosophy with everyone I encountered. I was truly feeling my oats.

Ah, yes, you could see it coming, couldn't you? The problem came in when I went home for Thanksgiving and discovered that if I reverted back to my old trick of eating fast, I could cram in more of my mother's cooking and my dad's apple pie before my stomach told me to stop. That would have been okay for one day, but once again, I found myself having to learn the hard way that I could never take a vacation away from self-control. The extremist in me can't handle a little leeway. It reverts back to its old habits with glee. It's almost as if my heart tagged me and yelled, "Gotcha!" and took off, dragging me back to every eating haunt that served a plate of my favorites. "Go ahead," my heart said. "You owe it to yourself," it cajoled. "You've been good for so long, you deserve a break today." The rest is pitiful; you know the drill—repeat history. Before I knew it, the twenty pounds I had lost returned and brought ten friends with it.

Unfortunately, I had mastered the Weigh Down technique without mastering my heart. Let me just say this. You can listen to your heart if you want to, but a heart that is not submitted and disciplined to do the right thing is not your friend. It will talk you into eating everything in sight, then turn around and despise you when you blow back up. It will criticize you and make you feel so bad about yourself you won't be able to find the strength you need to climb back up on the horse you fell off. Don't listen to an untrained heart. Take it from me, the voice of experience.

Think about it. Why do we call certain foods comfort food? How can food be a source of comfort? It can't tell you anything to fix your situation, so how much comfort does it really give? You have to be drunk on food for it to medicate you and make you feel better, which suggests you have to eat too much to get to this state. Ladies, what are we doing to ourselves? We have got to stop the madness, and it begins with getting our hearts in line with our minds. We cannot make food another bad man in our lives. We are going to take control of our love lives. We are going to love ourselves more than we love food and tear that idol right off the altar of our hearts.

We are going to crucify our heart attitudes about food once and for all. There will be no turning back. Don't expect your heart to give up its dominion of you peacefully. It will shriek like a vampire facing the sun, but I say ignore the noise and keep shining the light until you feel strong enough to stand on your new principles. So take a deep breath and repeat after me: *Losing weight does not have to be that deep, but it does begin with me making a decision to permanently change my attitude and my heart toward food and how I eat it—and that is a good thing.*

Girl, your hips are going to love you for it!

KEEPING IT REAL

- Keep track of your emotions as they relate to food for one week.

- What does your heart tell you about food when you are happy? sad? angry? stressed? bored? content?

- When and why do you eat? Do you ever give thought to the size of your portions? What drives you to clean your plate?

- How do you feel after you have stuffed yourself? What vows do you make at the moment? Do you keep them? What makes you break them?

- How badly do you want to lose weight? What is really stopping you? What conversation do you need to have with yourself to get on the right path to permanent weight loss?

- Try listening to your body (that would be your stomach and your taste buds) vs. your heart for a week, and see if you can tell the difference.

DIVA REFLECTIONS

Stop beating yourself up. Low self-esteem and self-degradation are counterproductive to losing weight or doing anything good for yourself. For every day that you lose ground in your war with your weight, there is another day for gaining back the ground you lost. Take it one day at a time, and make the decision not to allow long lapses of self-control. There is something to be said for rewarding yourself for small victories, but even the *Emmy Awards* go off at ten o'clock (11 p.m. eastern standard time)! Can you imagine an award show going on for days and days? People would say, "Enough already," and stop watching. Girl, get a grip on yourself! Rewards are meant to be short acknowledgments for a job well done, not an unending soliloquy. Keeping things in perspective is a major part of the battle won with your heart. You can do it!

7

Attitude Check

THE REASON YOU HAVE got to take control of your heart condition is because your heart will rule your attitude. I'll say it again—attitude is everything. Attitude affects your emotions, your focus, your beliefs, your response to what is happening or not happening in your life. Based on how you respond, your entire life can be affected. One bad choice is all it takes to ruin a promising life. One good choice is all it takes to kick open the door to endless, incredible possibilities.

So how do you feel about how you look right now? Are you depressed? resigned? ambivalent? nonchalant? angry? What are you? Whatever frame of mind you are in is going to determine how you treat yourself and your approach toward food. Food should be neither foe nor friend; it has no personality. It is something that is to be used to your advantage. So let's master food. I know that when you are salivating over a dish that looks delicious, it's easy to think that the food is controlling your appetite, but indeed, you are still very much in control. However, if you haven't made some decisions on what you are going to do about your weight, you will cave. You've got to have a plan.

This is why it is so important to renew our minds. It has a literal impact on whether we will experience transformation. We become what we believe. Remember that faith is contingent on what you are hoping for and what you believe will be. You will make choices based on what you believe. Those choices will have results or outcomes that will either confirm or disappoint your expectations, which will affect your response. That response will either solidify or destroy your faith and affect the next course of action you take. So the short of it all is, if you expect something and it doesn't happen, you'll say to yourself, "See, I knew it wouldn't work," and be reluctant to try again. This is what happens with most diets if you've been seesawing up and down the scale. You do well for a while, but then you implode and conclude that diets just don't work for you. You then give up altogether until you gain enough weight to become desperate enough to try another fad diet.

That's what I did with a series of short-term, drastic, quick-fix diets. Let's see, there was the cabbage diet, the rice diet, the lemonade diet. All of these diets are designed to take your body on a crash course of getting off ten pounds or more—just like that! C'mon! Nothing in life is "just like that." (Well, nothing intended to last longer than the one minute, one day, or one week it took to get it—you know what I'm talking about!) Only through the magic of television do people fall in love, become stars, bounce back from adversity, and turn from frogs into princes . . . just like that. And as predicted, those "just like that" diets worked . . . for the moment. In retrospect, I wonder how much I hated myself to torture my body like that. What kind of message was I sending to the rest of me? *All right, body. I am going to torture you, degrade you, and deny you until you line up and make me look beautiful.* No wonder my body hit me back with more weight than I had lost. It was the ultimate revenge designed to show me who was really in charge.

Furthermore, these quickie diets are a sure way to mess up your metabolism. I think a ruined metabolism is the body's way of telling you it doesn't trust you to take care of it anymore. You've starved it and left it to fend for itself so many times before that it decides to take matters into its own hands. So now, when you start drifting toward all those crazy combinations and varieties of starvation, your body sends out an alert to all parts: "All right, body parts. She's at it again. It's time to batten down the hatches. We've got to hold on to what we've got in case she never feeds us again! Who knows how long this one will last?" Notice that it gets harder to lose it each time? Mm-hmm. Now you know why.

So as Patti LaBelle sings, it's time to get a new attitude. Enough with the torture. I don't know about you, but I'm a happy sanguine. If something isn't fun, I don't want to do it. I (and other sanguines) think you get a whole lot more cooperation from folk if they feel they are making a contribution to what you're doing *and* if they enjoy what they are doing. So we are going to get our bodies to partner with us and enjoy the experience of losing weight together.

Well, how are we going to do that, Michelle? I hear you. I know you've been bogged down into thinking a diet is more like a dirge for so long that you can't even restructure your brain to think anything else right now, right? It's like being drafted to go to some remote place to fight where none of your usual comforts will exist. Uh-huh, that's why we hoard right before a diet. Can I get a witness? We decide that next week is the week. But up until then, it's on! We eat everything we think we will miss, and then some, to ramp up for the big day when the official denial begins. That is no way to win a war. That just sets you up to make a date to return back to all those things in greater volume once you conclude you've denied yourself long enough. Where is the balance?

It's like the single woman who views every man she meets as her potential husband. It's a setup for disappointment. Every man you meet is not going to be husband material or your husband.

However, he might be a good friend or even introduce you to the man who may be your husband, but you will never get that far if you eliminate each male because he personally doesn't want to get you to the altar or he isn't your "type." What am I saying? Life is not that black or white. Do or die. Or diet. There is a place in the middle where everyone can feel safe and make more organic choices for themselves.

In my journey toward holistic and permanent weight loss, I realized that I have to step back from how I view dieting and decide to make some long-term goals for myself and my body—goals that we can both live with for a lifetime. Consistency is going to be the key to permanently getting and keeping the results I want. So I'm going to take the courtship approach—slow and steady. I am going to avoid microwave love. (That's where things heat up fast and cool off even faster.) I am going to make peace with the fact that it took more than a week to put on all the weight I now carry and it will take more than a week to get it off. That is fair, and I'm sure your body will happily agree with me. So I'm going to take the rational approach to moving forward as I would with a new relationship.

First I'm going to think the best and see the potential. We can use the election phrase here rather effectively: "Yes, we can!" Failure is not an option. It is not possible because I'm running this. I am partnering with my body to be a better me. What a team! We can do this! Yes! Get enthusiastic about it. You're not going to a funeral. You're headed toward a better quality of life. There will be no expiration date. I am not going to rush this. I am going to realistically approach everything about my lifestyle and make some shifts that will enhance my life and my joy level. The side benefit will be that pounds will begin to melt away. My body will find the place that is comfortable for it and maintain its new, svelte self without coercion.

There. Doesn't that sound a whole lot better than *I'm going to starve myself and beat myself up until my body cooperates and drops the pounds in less than two weeks!?* I thought so. What were you thinking, girl? Your Guantánamo Bay is closed. It's official: You can end the torture. So join me and make the shift in your head. You are not going on any more diets. I find it interesting that the beginning of that word is *die*. Die to the word *diet*. We can choose to *die* to the things that are not working for us, and once we are refocused and have put those cravings to death, they won't resurrect or rise up to haunt us. A dead person has no reaction if you wave her favorite dish under her nose. Why? Because she is dead. She is no longer moved by any stimulus. She has left the building and gone on to, hopefully, a better life.

We all need to die, but no *one* or no *thing* should kill us. We have the privilege of choosing to lay our lives down; we can choose to lay our desires down and we can choose to pick them up again. In other words, we can take control of our lives by willingly submitting to what is best. Remember, the choice is yours. When you choose the path of denial, you give the power to the thing you are denying yourself of. You will keep thinking about it until you can have it again. But if you decide that you will either no longer partake of that thing or indulge in limited measures because your health is more important to you, the power is back in your hands. That should make you feel strong and joyful and keep you on track to a thinner, healthier you.

So there you have it. This book, regardless of its title, is not about a diet at all. It's all about you getting to the best part of you and staying there. So you have a decision to make. It's up to you to make the attitude shift. You are what you think. There is no room for being double minded. Your inner conflict will stall your results. A house or a body divided against itself will fall.[1] With great dreams comes great responsibility. Are you ready to take the helm and steer your ship/your life? Your decision is the ultimate power. I believe that God is bored with indecision. Actually I think it grieves Him. He can't help you if you can't make up your mind. So, take a deep breath. You can do this. One day at a time. Make the decision to go the distance. A new lifestyle is a journey, not a sprint. Decide to enjoy the sights along the way rather than think of what you might have missed. You'll be amazed at what you discover.

KEEPING IT REAL

Use the following questions and activities to be honest about your attitude toward dieting:

- Make a list of all the diets you've ever done before and their outcomes.

- Make a list of things that got you off track in each instance when you regained the weight. What was going on in your life? How did you feel emotionally? How did you respond?

- What mind shifts do you need to make toward how you view your body and take care of yourself?

- What new attitude do you need to develop toward food?

DIVA REFLECTIONS

Mind renewal can be an exhausting process. Your will must prevail. It has taken you a long time to believe what you believe. However, the brain cannot separate fact from fiction. Therefore, you get to create a new reality for yourself. Learn to use your mind in more powerful ways. Harness your imagination, and make it work for you. Picture the you that you want to see in the mirror. Capture that picture, and preserve it in your heart. If you can see it, you can attain it. Now endure the race for the prize you see looming before you. It is within reach.

8

From Your Lips to Your Hips

REMEMBER WHEN LADY O, as I am fond of calling Oprah, pulled a wheelbarrow onto the stage of her talk show after she lost all that weight the first time? The wheelbarrow was piled high with the amount of fat that she had lost. It was a shocking but effective visualization that showed there is a huge difference between an actual pound of fat and the small line on your bathroom scale. Somehow, looking at an incremental measure just doesn't do justice to the reality of what we are really dealing with. I remember thinking as I looked at the fat in the wheelbarrow, *That is just not possible. All that was not on girlfriend's body.* Ah, but indeed it was. A pound is a pound no matter how you look at it. Just because it's spread out between the top of your head and the tips of your toes doesn't mean that pound diminishes in some way.

So what are you looking at when you look at your body? I'm looking at sloppy joes around my midsection, that's what I'm looking at. Without the sauce. Go ahead. Go to the grocery store. Head straight to the meat section, and look at the ground beef. Look at what a pound looks like. Now calculate how much weight you want to lose and stack up that many pounds of hamburger and see what you get. (Sometimes you have to face the enemy head on, and it ain't pretty, my friend.)

As long as you romanticize your fat, you will never lose it. You've got to look at the ugly truth. Deal with it, sister! The "it's not that bad" syndrome has got to stop. It *is* that bad. High cholesterol, anyone? Hiding behind layers of clothing? Giving up on your appearance? Feeling a little slow and run down? It's only natural when you're carrying around extra poundage. You have to work harder to dress it up and get where you want to go. What you need is a little leverage to pop you out of your present state and propel you toward a better, healthier you.

So now, close your eyes—but not before you read what I tell you to do! After you close your eyes, I want you to imagine yourself the size you are now five years from now. Then add ten pounds to that image because we usually gain a few pounds per year as we get older. Imagine how you look and how you feel in five years (with this extra ten pounds). Think about yourself—not just physically but emotionally. Now think forward in time another five years, always adding another ten pounds for every five years until you just can't stand to think of yourself this size. What year did you get to, and how loud did you scream? Sometimes you have to see the big picture—literally, no pun intended. Now that you've seen where you don't want to go, decide where you *do* want to go.

But slow down! No need to go off the deep end and rush off on some crazy collision course of a crash diet. Just consider the word *crash*. That's exactly what you do—crash and burn—anytime you go to drastic measures to shock your body into losing weight. Remember, we are exercising discipline. Eating responsibly. Not starting habits we can't maintain.

Now that we've made some progress with our heart conditions and our attitudes, we have got to put our language—yes, the things we say—in check. Words have power. It's amazing that one little thing, namely our tongues, can accomplish such great deeds. It can literally set the world on fire. One person yells something out of fear, and everyone starts running. Buildings empty. Time stands still until another word releases us to return back to normal. One whispered sentence can make or destroy a person's life. Words float out into the atmosphere and gain momentum, which creates their own reality, whether they are true or not. This is why we must be careful about what we say of others and what we say about ourselves. You will literally become a prisoner of your own words. So guess what? The moment you declare, "I'm fat!" whether in jest or all sincerity, you've sealed your fate to remain in that condition. There is a thin line between your present reality and the reality you want to create. Look at the difference of saying this: "I may be overweight today, but this is a temporary state. Keep watching. Get ready to see a new me!"

So let's redo our vocabularies. We may not like the way we look right now, but that is no reason to repeat the obvious. We have affirmed the negative long enough to convince ourselves that this is the life we're destined to live. But that is not true unless we allow it to be. On these grounds, let's begin to speak solutions over ourselves. Remember, you can have what you say. Write it down, and it gains power. Have you ever noticed that all these weight-loss places—Weight Watchers, Jenny Craig, you name it—all ask you to keep a journal of what you are eating? I totally get it. If you have to write it down, maybe you won't eat it. But if you write it down, you can also see where you went wrong. It helps you keep track of your progress and makes you deal with any lies that you may have been telling yourself.

I don't know about you, but when I say, "I'm fat," I get depressed and go in search of something fattening to put in my mouth. My rationale? Why not? I'm already fat, so one more fattening thing is not going to hurt me at this point. But if I say, "I lost a pound this week," all of a sudden I don't want to mess up my progress. A friend of mine always signs off from our phone calls with, "I'm looking forward to seeing less of you!" To which I happily quip, "Me, too!" You see where I'm going with this? One set of words sends me down the exact opposite path of action—one toward more destruction, the other toward victory. Which one do you want to choose?

Patience with yourself is key when it comes to renovating your vocabulary. Cheerleaders don't stop cheering at a game when the opponent gets a point or their team fumbles the ball. As a matter of fact, they go into overdrive: "That's all right, that's okay, we're gonna beat you anyway!" Training yourself to recover and remain optimistic is important to winning any game. So now, besides writing down what you eat, you need to keep a victory journal. Chronicle your success; document how it makes you feel and what you anticipate for your life based on your progress.

Now, here's the biggie: We are no longer going to say we are on a *diet*. Just the word makes everything in your system go into rebellion and reach for the creamiest thing you can find. Remove every reference to denial and deprivation. This is about you making different personal choices. This is about you feeling empowered to choose something simply because you prefer to do something that is good for yourself. Don't set yourself up for others to try to tempt you and break your resolve. You know the minute you utter, "I'm on a diet," someone will always be there to rationalize your taking one bite. "One bite won't hurt you . . ." But when you say, "No, I don't care for that," no one is going to argue with that or try to make you believe otherwise! The moment you say, "I'm on a diet," you're doomed. And saying, "I'm on a diet," hints at not being a permanent arrangement, which defeats the goal of eating and living healthily for a lifetime. We've done the diets and bounced back the heftier for it. We are not playing that game anymore. What we are aiming for here is a nice balance of changing our eating habits and making healthier choices *joyfully*. We are taking our approach to eating out of our intellect alone and employing our emotions. Let's face it: Our emotions are a powerful driver. We're used to eating emotionally but for all the wrong reasons. So let's use our emotions for our positive good. We are eating differently because we *enjoy* eating differently, not because we have to. This is our goal. It is achievable. And it is so empowering to know that we are making the choice and not allowing our hearts to boss us around.

I had to make some choices when I found out that some things were giving me acid reflux. I love, love, love (did I say love?) orange juice. I hope you get how deeply I love OJ. But I can't drink it. The pain outweighs the pleasure. I have a choice. I can drink the juice and try to live with the awful feeling of acid reflux (not!); I can take medicine just to have a glass of orange juice (not ideal); or I can find an alternative that I enjoy just as much or more and kiss that orange juice fondly good-bye (sorry, but I've got to love you and leave you, as the French say!). The same choices hold true for whatever foods are not your friends. If you knew someone was an unrepentant mass murderer, would you hang out with that person, with the knowledge that he or she was capable of hurting you? Why do we compartmentalize choices in life? Whatever isn't good for you just is not good for you. It's just not smart to keep hanging out with folks who have a history of harming you, or staying in situations that are detrimental to your life, so why do we treat harmful food differently? Every now and then, I fondly reminisce about having a glass of orange juice, but my daydream is short lived when I recall that awful acid reflux burning sensation that feels like someone threw a match down my throat. The mere memory of the pain is enough to keep me on track. I don't have a problem with avoiding orange juice. It is my choice not to consume it. I am more focused on feeling good.

Just as I have learned to deal with my love of orange juice, your language and your focus has to shift so that you don't feel as if you are being held against your will. Remember, you are in control. Plus, it's very diva-esque to say, "I'm just not that hungry," or "You know, all of a sudden, I just l-o-o-ve asparagus!" All my thin friends just love all the things that go crunch while I hunt(ed) for the butter. But things have changed. I found out that the crunchy stuff makes you feel more full. And a little low-fat cream cheese goes a long way to ease my butter cravings. Aha, there's a silver lining in this thing. You just have to find it.

It's a powerful thing when your attitude gets married to your lips; it translates to your hips. You will begin to speak positive, life-giving statements over everything and see yourself begin to flourish. Remember, God created an entire universe with words. He spoke, and it was. As His children, we've inherited the same creative ability. This is why we must reign over our thought lives and focus on what is true, pure, and of a good report—all the things that give life.[1] 'Cause when the squeeze is on, whatever is in you is what will come out. The way you perceive things is what you will believe, speak, and act on. It's the glass is half-full or half-empty train of thought. Depending on what that means to you, your view of the contents can cause peace or angst and set off a specific set of actions that could be good or bad for you.

Your words are the reflection of your thoughts, beliefs, and attitudes. It's interesting that thunder is the sound that lightning makes, but that sound is usually delayed. We see the lightning first and hear the thunder later. By then the lightning has struck. Your attitude can cause damage before you say anything, but your words will definitely seal your fate in some instances, so be aware of what you are creating for yourself with your words. In light of this fact, let's decide to line up with this diva confession: "I am beautiful, I am fabulous, and I am on my way to an even better me." (And you know that D.I.V.A. is my acronym for Divine Inspiration for Victorious Attitude, right?!) So here's a high five, girlfriend! I'm standing with you, and there is a whole lot of power in agreement.

KEEPING IT REAL

- What have you been saying about yourself? How has that made you feel? How has it made you act?

- What self-defeating confessions have you gotten in the habit of blurting out "in jest"? Is there any truth behind the joke? Why do you say these things?

- What comments have others made that affect how you feel about yourself? How do you put those comments in perspective?

- How have words damaged you in the past? How have they affected your actions?

- What new truth can you select for yourself? Write down the new truth, and carry it around with you.

DIVA REFLECTIONS

My dog whisperer, Erdem, told me that I must never say my dogs' names in anger, frustration, or impatience. Their names are supposed to only be associated with affection and praise so that they always respond positively when I call. (Talk about the need to renew my mind.) My first impulse when they do something wrong is to yell their names. It took me a while to remember to just calmly say, "Hey! No!" Guess what? It works. It works with humans, too. What we say, the tone, and the timing all glean positive or negative responses. There is a difference between a slave and a willing servant. So be kind to yourself and your body. It will serve you well in the end.

What Have You Got to Lose?

I KNEW I WAS IN TROUBLE. My doctor had called and left a message on my voice mail, and she sounded serious. When I finally worked up the nerve to return the call, she gently voiced her concern about my cholesterol level. It was high—frighteningly high. I was on the brink of heart disease, if not a heart attack. That could have explained my bouts with shortness of breath and why I waddled like a beached whale after taking one flight of stairs. I looked at my fluffy midsection and decided it was time to get serious about taking the weight off. My doctor ordered me to take one of those cholesterol drugs. Can you say *Lipitor*? Now it just might be me, but I hate drugs—anything in pill form or any liquids. I also hate the idea of having to take a medication for the rest of my life. I just can't stick to that long of a commitment. I always start off so well, but by the time I'm halfway through the bottle, I've gotten distracted, and the rest is history until I go to clean out my pantry. You would think I run a small pharmacy with all the herbs, supplements, and remedies I have.

Well, remember the Daniel fast I told you about in chapter 4? I decided to do it again and cleanse my system first. Sure enough, when I went back to the doctor for my second cholesterol test, the numbers had dropped significantly. The nurse was literally vibrating through the phone when she called to tell me, "So what we want to do next is adjust your prescription." I practically crowed, "Well, to be perfectly honest, I didn't take the medication." I heard a sharp intake of breath. "What did you do?" she asked. I told her all about how I had been eating. She was impressed but not convinced that I didn't still need to medicate myself and cautioned me to that end. I listened but decided I didn't want to be in bondage to a little white pill every day just because I couldn't shut my mouth or eat the right things. WARNING: Do not try this at home and then try to sue me if it doesn't work for you. The body is an individual and finicky thing. What works for one may not work for the other. I am not your doctor; I am simply trying to illustrate a basic principle here.

The basic principle is that in a lot of cases, we truly are what we eat. I believe most of our health issues can be solved by adjusting our eating habits. When we do eat right, not only do we lose weight, but we lose a lot of other things that threaten our joy, peace, and overall state of well-being. My cholesterol's going down was not the only health change I noticed when I did my Daniel fast. Prior to my cleansing, I had bloated ankles and sore feet. Whenever I got up from a chair, it was as if all the bones in my feet had to resettle before I could walk away. I ached. My knees hurt. I was always tired. I felt old—far older than I should have felt.

As the sugar and sodium left my system, so did all these ailments. My cholesterol went down. I felt great! The other thing I found interesting was that I wasn't as averse to exercise because I had more energy. When I exercised, all my endorphins kicked in big time. I was feeling good and looking even better. Girl, you couldn't tell me anything. In all honesty I knew that cholesterol would probably be a constant battle for me. Beyond my diet, I was affected by genetics and stress. Both of my parents had high cholesterol and heart disease, so I would always have to take extra care in this area.

Speaking of stress, I noticed this was another area that was affected when I took control of what I ate. I seemed more even tempered and less volatile. My mood swings mellowed to a more manageable place. In the light of the fact that I was premeno-pausal, this was a major miracle.

Why do I bring all this up? Because you need all the leverage and the reasons you can get to solidify your commitment to do the right thing by your body. Your first inclination to diet could be based on pure cosmetics. Perhaps you've pulled some photo of an unrealistic beauty out of a magazine and decided you want to look like her so you could wear the dress she had on. Trust me, after many years of being an art director in the advertising world, I can tell you that no one really looks like that photo. Only after hours of makeup, hairstyling, and manipulating of lights do many of those touted as the most beautiful women in the world emerge as the vixens we believe they are. Then, after all of that, let's not even discuss the retouching and the power of a single click and computer mouse to enhance, plump up, slim down . . . do you get my drift? Ah, if only life were so simple and my thighs were only a mouse click away from being free of cellulite and a few inches. The long and short of it is that beauty fades no matter how fabulous you are. Health is just more important than looking good—'cause if you keel over from a heart attack or are careening out of control because of sugar highs, your beauty—or lack of beauty—will mean nothing. Truly external factors cannot be the only reason you choose to get serious about what you are eating.

So let's talk about what else you have to lose from the inside out. I think the biggest thing that affects our beauty is our mental and emotional state. Depression can disfigure the most beautiful of the beautiful. Lots of foods can contribute to this—quite unbeknownst to us. Read the book *Sugar Blues* by William Dufty, and you may decide to curtail your sweets, sweetie. In addition to contributing to obesity and chronic disease, sugar causes drastic peaks and valleys in the chemical makeup of your system that can account for mood and energy swings. While you're blaming your depression on the weight, you might need to blame it on the sugar. Sugar and fat can be a bad mixture that can cause your spirits to spiral downward. Talk about the garment of heaviness![1] How about what your garments can do to your innards if they're too tight? I remember when one of my boyfriends asked if he could look in my closet. I gave him permission. He held up a hand and said quite dramatically, "Wait! Before I open this door, I want to illustrate what I think your clothes look like in this closet." He stood upright, squeezed his arms as closely to his sides as he could, and scrunched up his face; he then used this small voice to say, "Wait, can you scoot over a little? I'm scrunched, I can't breathe . . ." insinuating that my clothes were all crammed into a space too small to contain them. I laughed until tears streamed down my face. He was right. My closet was jam-packed, and my clothes had nowhere to go. Now, I could use that same picture for our organs. When you're the right size for your frame, your organs can breathe and cohabit in the right position or space. But when you are carrying extra pounds, or baggage as I like to call it, your vital organs are cramped, and they make you hurt. When I lose weight, I breathe more easily. My posture is better. I'm not bowed over, experiencing aches and pains, because everything is aligned as it should be. Don't you want to feel like that? I thought you did.

There are some other factors we don't think about when it comes to our health and our eating habits. What does all that weight do to your social life because of how you view yourself? How does it affect your self-esteem? your love life? your social interactions? Have you become a hermit? antisocial? or an awkward wallflower when you do venture forth? Do you spend time envying smaller women or concluding like the comedienne Mo'Nique that "skinny women are evil"? Is every woman who you consider to be more attractive than yourself a potential foe or friend because of how you feel about yourself? Most women have a hard time celebrating other women when they feel bad about themselves. Jealousy and envy will always create strife, gossip, and all kinds of needless chaos. So don't be a hater. It's time to kiss fat ankles, achy joints, high cholesterol, high blood pressure, acid reflux, diabetes, bad skin, a stunted social life (shall I go on?) . . . good-bye! Get to work on yourself, girl, 'cause you've got more than inches to lose and a whole lot of self-esteem and better health to gain!

KEEPING IT REAL

- You won't need the mirror for this one. How do you feel? Mentally? Physically?

- How do you feel about women who are the size you want to be?

- How does your present size affect how you relate to other women? men? yourself?

- What type of medications are you on? How would a change of diet affect your health?

- What commitment will you make to yourself right now to set you on the path to a healthier you?

DIVA REFLECTIONS

Committing is never the issue with most people when it comes to dieting. It is our ability to remain committed to our commitments. Therefore, make realistic goals and adjustments in your diet that you can stick to. Remember, we are dying to the concept of "diet."

Every move we make from now on is a permanent change in life. This way we don't bite off more than we can chew, no pun intended. Start with cutting one thing out of your diet and sticking with that until you don't miss it, then move on to the next. Choose some new healthy foods you hadn't considered trying. Experiment and find healthy replacements for some of the things you enjoyed that don't serve your body well. Baby steps. Hey, it took a long time to pile on the weight, so now be patient. Remember, the race is not won by the swift but by those who endure to the end.[2]

Going Nowhere Fast

HOW HAVE I LOST WEIGHT? Let me count the ways and the weigh-ins over the years! A diet by any other name is still a diet. And to be honest, they all work . . . for the time you're on them. Uh-huh, I hope you're getting this. Don't you just love it when folks promise you that you will lose ten pounds in two days? Now think about how that sounds, ladies. And yet we get sucked in every time. I can't tell you how many pills and potions I have purchased that promised to trim down my waistline, remove stubborn fat that refused to go anywhere, reduce cellulite . . . who are they kidding? Us—that's who! We're the ones buying their promises, hook, line, and sinker. Don't be a silly fish. That ten pounds lost in two days will soon turn into twenty pounds gained in four days—just as soon as you stop taking those pills or drinking only lemon and water; you know you can't live like that for long.

How long did it take you to put on that weight? What makes you think you can take off those same pounds in what would seem like milliseconds in comparison? Forget about it. Those pounds have settled in and taken up residence. They are comfortable. They have taken their shoes off and put their feet up and committed to sitting a while (if not permanently). If you try to rush them out of the house, they'll just be back, claiming they forgot something. When you have squatters, you have to be way more strategic in how you get rid of them once and for all. You've got to trick them into thinking they are going willingly. There is no other way to get the pounds off and keep them off. So settle in, sister. Realistically speaking, if you want to keep the pounds off, you are going to have to take them off slowly. Your fat has a long memory. You are going to have to make it forget where it was living, so embrace the process and settle in for the long haul. Hopefully, by the time you arrive at your destination, your entire outlook on food, your body, and how you live your life will have been so transformed that there's no way that fat can come back—it won't be able to find an open door. Don't be deceived; what a woman sows, she will also reap.[1] So, if you are into the yo-yo syndrome of losing weight quickly and wondering how all that fat found its way back to your thighs, quickly pull up a chair, and let's hash this out once and for all.

I remember many years and pounds ago when my friend Sandra and I decided to do the cabbage diet. It was so long ago that all I have is a vague remembrance of making this cabbage soup with lots of onions. We spiced it up really well, and it was actually rather yummy. We had this soup with different combinations of low-fat, low-calorie, and low/no sugar food every day for a seven-day period. I guess the food combinations were supposed to jolt your metabolism and system into behaving and burning all the fat in your body faster than normal. But basically it was really a modified fast. Low calories and no sugar or fat were the key to this diet causing you to lose ten to fifteen pounds in a week. You heard me, sister! Yes, I said up to fifteen pounds in one week. Unbelievable! I could sign up for that, if I only had to torture myself for seven days. Having a partner in crime totally helped. So

I camped out at Sandra's house, and we cooked up a major batch of soup and hunkered down to lose weight together.

Here's a sample cabbage soup diet plan[2] (you can find several other variations online):

DAY 1: Cabbage soup and all the fruit you want except bananas. Drink unsweetened tea, black coffee, cranberry juice, or water.

DAY 2: Cabbage soup, all the low-calorie vegetables you want (except beans, peas, or corn), and a baked potato with butter

DAY 3: Cabbage soup and a mixture of the above fruit and vegetables

DAY 4: Cabbage soup, up to eight bananas, and two glasses of skim milk

DAY 5: Cabbage soup; up to twenty ounces of beef, chicken, or fish; up to six fresh tomatoes; and at least six to eight glasses of water

DAY 6: Cabbage soup, up to three beefsteaks, and unlimited vegetables

DAY 7: Cabbage soup, up to two cups of brown rice, unsweetened fruit juices, and unlimited vegetables

The recipe for the cabbage soup varies slightly among different versions of the diet. But it basically includes cabbage and assorted low-calorie vegetables, such as onions and tomatoes, and is flavored with onion soup mix, bouillon, and tomato juice.

Here's a basic recipe:

- 1 celery stick (not the whole stalk), diced
- 3 carrots, sliced
- 2 bell peppers, sliced

- 6 large green onions, or 1 large yellow, white, or purple onion, diced
- ½ head green cabbage, diced
- 12 cups water
- 2 bouillon cubes, either chicken or beef
- 1 package dry onion soup mix
- Salt, pepper, parsley, garlic powder, and soy sauce to taste (or any other seasoning you like)
- 2 cans of tomatoes, diced or whole

Spray a large pot with cooking spray and sauté all vegetables except cabbage and tomatoes until tender. Add cabbage and about twelve cups of water. Add bouillon cubes, soup mix, and seasonings. Cook until cabbage reaches desired tenderness. Add tomatoes.

It was yummy, but it also had a rather odorous effect—if you get where I'm coming from. So if you decide to try it, only hang out with those who love you and understand that bodily functions are a reality in life.

The cabbage soup was supposed to make you feel full, right? Wrong. Just the idea that I was doing a diet made me hungry. I got bored quickly with my limited list of "can haves." I constantly thought about what I was going to eat and when I could eat next. And I had a list in my head of what I would eat the moment I was finished losing my weight. I was dying to eat something with cheese on it. Get it? Dying . . . but not in the right way. Anyway, the cabbage soup diet did work. I proudly went out and bought several new outfits to celebrate my new, svelte self. And now that I was cute, I thought I could eat all the foods I missed while I was ladling the cabbage soup. Ah, famous last bites. All that rapid weight loss was primarily fluids, not fat. Before long, I was back to my original weight. But it didn't stop there. I added on an additional five pounds. At that point, even the clothes I'd had before didn't fit properly.

Next there was the rice diet. You guessed it. On this diet, I ate rice with everything. Hey, quit your whining! I was promised that I could lose twenty to thirty pounds in a month! I would move to China or Japan for that payoff. Being West Indian and West African, I was all in for the rice thing. This would be a piece of cake . . . er, or a kernel of rice. I bought a big sack of jasmine rice and prepared for a rice-in. It seemed simple enough. The end was in sight. In a month, I would be fabulous, and the torture would be worth it. Here's a basic breakdown of what I endured. Of course, I was responsible for counting calories and selecting the fruits and vegetables that were not loaded with calories and sugar. So things like the melon family were a staple, along with a cup of rice, or cottage cheese. You get the picture.

PHASE 1 — ONE WEEK

DAY 1

2 starches and 2 fruits at breakfast, lunch, and dinner

DAYS 2-7

BREAKFAST: 1 starch, 1 fruit, 1 nonfat dairy

LUNCH AND DINNER: 3 starches, 3 vegetables, 1 fruit

PHASE 2 — ONE WEEK

DAY 1

2 starches and 2 fruits at breakfast, lunch, and dinner

DAYS 2-6

BREAKFAST: 1 starch, 1 fruit, 1 nonfat dairy

LUNCH AND DINNER: 3 starches, 3 vegetables, 1 fruit

DAY 7

   BREAKFAST: 2 starches, 1 fruit

   LUNCH: 3 starches, 3 vegetables, 1 fruit

   DINNER: 3 starches, 3 protein (or 2 dairy), 3 vegetables, 1 fruit

PHASE 3 — MAINTENANCE

Same as phase 2, adding about two hundred more calories per week, until you stop losing weight.

DAY 1

   2 starches and 2 fruits at breakfast, lunch, and dinner

DAYS 2-5

   BREAKFAST: 1 starch, 1 fruit, 1 nonfat dairy

   LUNCH AND DINNER: 3 starches, 3 vegetables, 1 fruit

DAYS 6-7:

   BREAKFAST: 2 starches, 1 fruit

   LUNCH: 3 starches, 3 vegetables, 1 fruit

   DINNER: 3 starches, 3 protein (or 2 dairy), 3 vegetables, 1 fruit[3]

The rice diet also worked. But of course! I was only getting about between eight hundred and one thousand calories a day. That left a whole lot of room for hunger; and there wasn't enough variety to make me forget that I was starving myself. This diet bored me to tears, but I was determined! And, I was in a contest with a friend to see who would lose the most weight. I won! I won! I ran back to the closet to squeeze myself into my long-neglected "I'm keeping this until I lose weight" stash. I looked hot, but I never wanted to see rice again. I wanted to see everything else I was missing. I saw, and I ate. This time it didn't take as long as before to gain back the weight. It came back faster, bigger, and better than before. I added ten pounds to my original weight when I stopped this diet. I made sure I took pictures before I let that happen, though. I wanted to have proof that I had lost so much weight.

I have to admit, after bouncing back from the rice diet, I called a time-out from dieting for a while and just settled into my new but not really improved hefty status. I decided that if I had to die one day, I could at least enjoy everything I ate along the way. *Who said everybody in America had to look like a clothing rack anyway?* I convinced myself. Last I heard, some men liked a little meat on their bones, and I aimed to please. Sounded like a good justification to me. My apathy and self-delusion caused me to wallow in my opinion until I became bigger than I could stand. One of my mentors said, "Hey, what's going on with you, Missy? You're in the public eye; you've got to get your act and your body together!" *True dat*, I thought. But at this point, I was well off my game. I didn't know where or how to begin to get back on top of my weight. I felt like a hippo was sitting on my chest and I couldn't budge.

Enter Beyoncé Knowles stage right, looking thin, absolutely flawless, and gorgeous as ever (just when I concluded there was no room for improvement with her), telling Oprah how she dropped twenty pounds in no time flat for her new movie *Dreamgirls*. Beyoncé said she had done the master cleanse lemonade diet. Supposedly, disc jockey Howard Stern's assistant also lost seventy pounds on this. I pictured millions of women scampering to the store in search of lemons. I decided I had better get a move on before the country declared a shortage. Off to Whole Foods I went. Sure enough, they even had a pamphlet and all the ingredients ready and waiting. Obviously, the rush had been on, and I was on the late show. But better late than never! I mixed up my concoction and jumped into the pool.

Not only was the master cleanse supposed to help you lose weight, but it was supposed to have many healing effects on the body, all of which I could use. It was supposed to flush from your body all the internal waste that clogs up your colon. The cleanse could even wash out gallstones, which are supposedly deposits of cholesterol that accumulate (I had never heard that before). It was also supposed to normalize your appetite and restore your metabolism, cleanse and detox your entire body, cleanse and restore your glandular system, and restore suppressed hormone levels (although I didn't know if I needed to feel any sexier, since I was a single woman trying to live holy). The list of the things the cleanse could do went on—it could reduce internal inflammation and boost your energy levels. Wow! Who would have thought that a handful of lemons could do all that?!

One doctor was quoted as saying that our bodies become so polluted with the toxins we ingest that they start to seep through the walls of our bowels, enter the bloodstream, and slowly poison us from the inside, something he called "autointoxication." Ew! It reminded me of the time I got alcohol poisoning as a teenager after a night of striving to prove how much vodka and orange soda I could hold. To this day, I'm not sure who really won that contest. But I remember being so ill that I wanted my mommy even though she would have finished me off if she had seen me that way. So I called for Jesus instead, although I didn't really know Him or think He would approve of my little adolescent drinking binge either. I just figured He would be kinder. So with this picture of what I was possibly doing to my insides, I committed to sticking it out with this cleanse. Here's what I had for ten days:[4]

Lemonade Diet

For at least ten days, drink around ten servings per day of the following:

- 2 tablespoons (1 fluid ounce) fresh-squeezed organic lemon or lime juice, NOT BOTTLED JUICE (approx. ½ lemon)

- 2 tablespoons (1 fluid ounce) organic Grade B maple syrup
- ⅒ teaspoon or more cayenne pepper (hot red pepper)
- 1 cup (8 fluid ounces) purified or spring water, NOT fluoridated water.

Shake it all up. This makes one serving!

Saltwater Flush
First thing in the morning, drink a mixture of

- 2 level teaspoons of uniodized sea salt and
- 1 quart of lukewarm water

Herbal Laxative Tea
You can find herbal laxative tea at most grocery stores (I used Smooth Move Tea). Each evening drink an herbal laxative tea to help with elimination—preferably right before bed.

That's it! No food. Just the concoctions listed above. Do that for at least ten days for a complete intestinal cleanse.

I did lose some weight after my cleanse, but not as much as Beyoncé. I caved. I could not keep going. I developed severe acid reflux. The thought hadn't occurred to me that if I couldn't do orange juice, I couldn't do lemon juice, either. They are both acidic, too acidic for my system. So while I enjoyed the benefits of doing a good fast that also cleansed, the price was too high for my esophagus. My sister tried it and caved short of the third day. I tried to tell her that if she could make it past the third day, it would be smooth sailing, but she said she was getting too evil, having chills, and feeling nauseated. So I released her from her self-imposed torture; I told her it was okay to quit because a woman has to do what a woman has to do to maintain her sanity, especially if she wants to keep her job and family. So kudos to those who have tried it, fought the good fight and won is all

I have to say. You are a better woman than I am. Of course, the little weight I did lose from the cleanse came back and brought relatives and friends.

Obviously, the quick fix was not working for me. I was learning the hard way that quick victories did not lead to sustained peace in the war for my body. Nothing changed—only my dress size for a short period of time. I also confused my system; it no longer was sure if it should process my food and get rid of it or store the food in case I chose to put it on lockdown again. I made my body angry at me. My body stopped working with me. I was hurting it. It did not feel the love. So every time I went on a crash diet, my body fought back by snatching any fat I chose to share with it and hoarding it to get revenge. I was sure of it. I had a hip uprising going on, and I was losing the battle of the bulge. I think my thighs had meetings at night to discuss how to take me down. I would look bigger the next morning when I got up—that's the truth, and I'm sticking to it.

Reluctantly I had to conclude that a permanent fix was going to take more time than these ten-day crash diets and cleanses. Perhaps, if I took my time to take off the weight in a balanced manner, my body would forgive me and cooperate more. And you know, it's happening even as I write this book. But I'm not done with the story yet.

KEEPING IT REAL

- Make a list of all the crash diets you've ever been on. Write down the outcome of each one.

- How much weight have you gained from your first diet to now? How long did you maintain your weight loss between diets? How much more did you gain back?

- What food(s) made you relapse? Which specific foods are your weakness?

- What is your pattern of dieting? Do you binge before or after or both?

- What things can you put in place to help you stop the yo-yo effect?

DIVA REFLECTIONS

Nothing beats a good try better than a failure. It will convince you that nothing will ever work out for you. It will make you think that you are a loser, blah, blah, blah. Not true. Not true. At least you acknowledged that something was wrong and tried to do something about it. That puts you in a good position to have some success. Take the time to regroup, recover, learn from your mistakes, and move on. Be honest with yourself about what didn't work for you. Go easy. Your heart has to work harder when you stress it out with all these radical weight swings. Now is not the time to be impatient. You need to get your body to cooperate with you gladly and willingly. It was the turtle who won the race. Remember that. The hare is still shocked about it.

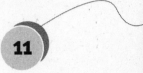

The Truth about Fasting

NOW THAT WE'VE TAKEN a look at all the masochistic things you can do to your body to punish it for not looking the way you want it to, it's time to reassess and put some things in perspective. First of all, it is not your body's fault that it is in the shape it is in. Let's unpack that for a second. Your body does not force you to eat what you eat or to do what you do or don't do. Your body is not the boss of you. You are the boss of it.

If I can lean back on my dog training for a moment, I'd like to make another point. When I act like the alpha dog or the one in charge, my dogs obey me. When I am a wishy-washy pack leader, they become ambivalent followers. They know they don't have to obey me; they test me and ignore me! Can you imagine? I have to remind them who fills their bowls and what side their bread or treat is buttered on. Anyway, the principle for eating healthily is that *you* are the master of your body, and it responds to your lead. If you choose to feed it good things, it will take them, ingest them, break them down, and process them without complaining. If you throw junk into your body, it will take that, too. It may burp, or do other unpleasant things that it cannot control, but that is your fault because of what you chose to feed it.

You can create habits that set your body up to crave all the bad things you've been giving it, thus leading to the rationale that your body is telling you what it wants, but that is not really true. Your body follows your lead. It can't wrestle you to the floor and force stuff down your throat. When you eat properly, your body begins to crave good things.

At this point in my life, I know when my system needs a break, because I will only desire some fruit or a great salad. I will actually crave some carrots or salsa or just some herbal tea. When I'm low on iron, I crave red meat. It's not my first choice to eat red meat, so I know that, when I have that craving, I'm missing something that my system needs. That's a safe lead that I can follow. I listen to my body the same way I listen to a good friend. Even good friends may sometimes give bad advice, but in those moments I still have the power to decide if what they are suggesting is good for me or not and make the right choice. I'm not going to give in to my body's every whim for Dairy Queen chocolate-dipped ice cream cones or Kit Kat bars, or Red Vines licorice, or gummy bears or . . . okay, I'd better stop! I can't go there! But you get the picture.

Your body is like a confused man. You know how we do the men, ladies. We tell them to be strong, to be sensitive. Take the lead; let me do it! They don't know what we want, so they abdicate altogether and do nothing. Then we get impatient with them, but that's another book. All I'm saying is that, to be consistent, act as if you are in control, and your body will line up and work with you to reach and sustain your goal.

Second, fasting is a good thing, but not for the wrong reasons. If I had chosen any of those fasts or quick-start diets from the previous chapter for the right reason, I would have been able to stay on track to losing weight. The right reason for quickie diets is to give you a jump start so that you see losing pounds is possible. This should encourage you to keep going with a modified, less drastic plan until you reach your goal. Hopefully between the fast and your healthy-eating plan, your eating habits have changed so much that there is no such thing as celebratory binges that set you right back where you came from. If you do major bingeing before starting a diet or a fast, that is your first indicator that you have lost the battle before you've even begun to fight the war. How you begin is how you will finish, which is why, sure as you are born, you binge again after you've lost the weight.

So what are the right reasons and the right way to fast? I'm glad you asked. I believe it is important to fast every now and then. I know some people who do a regular fast. One lady I know fasts every Monday. That is the day she has set aside to just realign herself and find her center, as she puts it. She says it's crucial to her being in command of her week. Another friend fasts every three months for seven days. I used to begin every year with a twenty-one-day liquid-only fast. *Why*, you say? This was my time of consecration. It was not about losing weight; it was my time of setting myself apart spiritually and realigning myself with God in order to get direction for the coming year. As I grew older, it became harder to do this, so I had to shorten the period of fasting, but I believe He honors it just the same. So there you have it. The right reason for fasting is twofold. First, it gives your system a chance to rest and cleanse itself. Imagine a garbage disposal that was being overwhelmed with garbage constantly being fed into it faster than it could process it. At some point, the garbage disposal would either become severely backed up or the motor would burn out from attempting to break everything down and dispose of it. But when it has had time to clear out everything that is in it, the process of elimination becomes more efficient. Same thing with the body. After a fast, your body is cleaner, and your organs have had the time to flush and rejuvenate themselves. The colon gets nice and clean because it has the time to finally eliminate whatever has been backed up in its upper space. You've seen people with distended stomachs. All of that is uneliminated waste, backed-up food that never got broken down and eliminated, just sitting there . . . ew! When you do a good cleanse, the stuff that comes out looks scary. If your body is functioning properly, you should eliminate up to five times a day or at least shortly after every time you eat. Sorry to get gross, but this is a reality you must face. The longer waste has been sitting in your intestines, the blacker and scarier it looks. A good cleanse that you can pick up at the health food store or the master cleanse, if you can handle the acid, will help you eliminate the garbage and toxins that could be stressing your entire system. These toxins are responsible for acid indigestion and reflux, making you sluggish, tired, sleepy, grouchy, slow on your feet, and even slower mentally. Am I pushing any buttons here? The wrong foods and uneliminated waste are the culprits. Stop beating up your body; it's doing the best it can to deal with what you're doing to it. It's like forcing a small horse to lug an ocean liner onto the shore in deep sand; it's just too much weight to pull. Everything is working against its being successful. It can only mark time at best; it can't do it. Small wonder, after a fast your acumen is actually stronger. Even your brain feels freer to function, and everything in your system is primed to be sharper. Make sense? An unclogged drain becomes an expressway for everything to function better and come out all right. Can I get an amen for starting a new movement?! Aha!

That being said, I now want to focus on the spiritual element of fasting. I believe that all human beings are triune beings in a sense. We are spirits that have souls that live in our bodies. You cannot ignore any part, or the entire body will be affected. This is what true holistic living is—nurturing your body, soul, and spirit.

In light of that, it is important to understand that whatever you feed is what will be the strongest.

The flesh is always at war with the spirit. The spirit is naturally attuned to God and wants to do things according to how it was originally programmed before we got involved with influencing it wrongly and allowing external stimuli to distract us from our original purpose. I think the process is kind of like a computer that runs at optimum performance until you start downloading a whole lot of programs that are in conflict with its operating system. You then have to clean off those programs to get your computer back to the way it was designed to run. Fasting forces your flesh to submit to the spirit; fasting silences the flesh's voice. Fasting strengthens your spirit so that it can once again clearly hear God's voice, discern His instruction, and master the flesh to follow God's lead. Whenever I have fasted, I have experienced amazing breakthroughs in my life and circumstances. It's as if my eyes are opened, although I thought they were open before. It's like the light comes on and all of a sudden I see what I didn't see before. I get clarity on issues and decisions; I seem to get wisdom about what I am supposed to be doing that leads to the outcome I was struggling so hard to reach before. I seem less resistant to letting go of the things I can't control, which makes room for things to fall into place with less struggle. Losing weight is the last thing on my mind during this time of fasting. This time is all about me getting my spirit attuned to get the victory I need in my life and relationships. Losing a few pounds is just an added perk.

The disciples asked Jesus in the Gospels why they were having such a hard time helping the people that came to them for deliverance, and Jesus told them that, in some cases, certain things could only be removed by fasting and prayer.[1] These were stronger devils that had to feel the full impact of a strong spirit in order to be shattered and give way to the other side of a person's struggles.

And so it is with us. Sometimes your fight is not just a natural one; sometimes it is spiritual. You have to fortify all fronts of your inner and outer being.

Sometimes our hunger is more spiritual than we know, so we keep eating without getting satisfied. Stop and listen. Jesus Himself said that we don't live by just the food or bread we put in our mouths but by every Word that comes out of the mouth of God. This suggests that God Himself feeds us when we seek Him. His words are a meal that can fill and satisfy us! One of my favorite Scriptures is when God calls out to the people in the book of Isaiah 55:2-3: "Why spend your money on food that does not give you strength? Why pay for food that does you no good? Listen to me, and you will eat what is good. You will enjoy the finest food. Come to me with your ears wide open. Listen, and you will find life" (NLT). Another translation says, "Hearken diligently unto me, and eat ye that which is good, and let your soul delight itself in fatness" (KJV). Thank God something can be fat!

During my years of struggling with my weight, I was trying to hear God, but I was too full! Too full of food and too full of myself. My ears were clogged. The sound of food digesting, pride, angst, my own agenda, you name it—it all drowned out the still, small voice of God's Spirit trying to communicate with mine and show me the way through the journey of this thing we call life. Remember the story of Daniel and his friends that I mentioned in chapter 4? If you recall, after they did their modified fast/diet, they not only looked physically better, but they were sharper mentally and seemed to possess greater wisdom and spiritual acumen—down to interpreting dreams and having prophetic vision—than their counterparts. Daniel and his boys were the ones who stood in the face of opposition and triumphed.

Daniel, in particular, became widely respected and known not only as a man of prayer but as a wise counselor to four Babylonian kings. Now, you know it's a major miracle for anyone in government to survive and be promoted through four administrations; and it's downright supernatural when you consider that he opposed most of their beliefs. I believe that for most of us, weight loss and healthy living are one of those things that cannot be achieved by natural strength alone. You need wisdom from on high, and the only way you can tap into the deeper recesses of God's heart and mind is by first emptying yourself and getting into the position to receive. When we are full of ourselves, we are not teachable or open to correction or direction. It's called humbling ourselves. And sometimes when we are hungry and our flesh is depleted, we are more open to this concept.

Practically speaking, you can choose your own kind of fast. There are tons of them that people do, and only you know what is a real sacrifice for you. Fasts range from no television or candy, for whatever time frame you decide, to no solid food. Because we're talking about food, I am going to focus there. You can do water only, liquids only, fruit and vegetables only—again, it's your choice. You can choose to fast half a day—from 6 a.m. to 6 p.m.—for a full day, three days, a week, up to forty days, or doing a modification week to week. (Example: The first week you do water or liquids only, the second week you consume some sort of broth that has a liquefied vegetable, the third week eat fruit only, fourth week fruit and vegetables, and after you break the fast, add in grains only for a few days and then small portions of meat to allow your system to readjust to all foods.) This is between you and God and your physician. Again, don't try this stuff and then write me to complain. You know your body and should always check with your doctor to make sure you are in condition to do a fast. I do think it's safe to say that no one has ever died or gotten sick from eliminating fried chicken from her diet, so don't run up a doctor's bill for stuff that just makes sense.

Know that your body will not wrap its arms around denial gladly, especially if your system is backed up and loaded down with toxins. It will fight you. Initially, you might get headaches; you might feel weak, nauseous, grouchy, irritable, and basically terrible as your body starts unearthing stuff it didn't know was still in it. Don't worry; you will survive and feel the better for fighting it out and showing your body who is boss.

You can prepare your body not to have to go through such severe withdrawal by doing some prep work before you begin your fast. Take an herbal laxative tea at night for three nights before you begin so that your body can begin to do some initial flushing before your empty stomach shows your system all the junk that's still left in it. Also start eating light three days before so that you're not adding to the backlog of things for your system to process. After all is said and eaten, your body will thank you for it like a child who finally grows up and understands what her parents were saying once she has children of her own. And guess what? You won't die even if it feels like it. There are people who go for much longer periods of time without food who are still here to tell their stories.

A fast reveals things about yourself and exposes idols in your life—things you would never have thought existed. It is amazing the things that become magnified when food isn't in the way! All the issues you've buried rise to the surface and demand answers. And the answers you've been avoiding become crystal clear. Hey, it's all a good thing in the name of making progress in life and love. As they say, if you want to get on with your life and get a better grasp of how to go about it, turn down your plate, open your Bible, and turn up your hands in prayer.

Purpose to listen more than you talk, and see what happens. It's kind of like the recipe for getting rid of a cold, which is simply a buildup of toxins and the body's way of expelling them. *Cough, sneeze, just get it out of me,* is what your body is saying.

Feed a cold, starve a fever. Starve your flesh, feed your spirit. The stronger one will win. There is a spiritual element to every area of our lives, including the hold that food can have on us. The bottom line? Some things are just not going to change for you until you choose to be the master of your body. And that, my friend, is the gospel truth.

KEEPING IT REAL

- Commit to a fast you can handle. Start with a one-day fast from 6 a.m. to 6 p.m.
- Prepare for the fast by eating light for three days. The night before your fast, don't eat anything after 6 p.m.
- Decide if you need to do your fast on a day when you don't have a lot of activity. (I personally think it is best to take a day to be quiet.)
- Don't tell anyone you are fasting or draw attention to it. The more that you focus on it, the harder it will be.
- Read your Bible or another book that feeds your spirit at mealtimes to replace your meal.

DIVA REFLECTIONS

Some of the things we war with in life cannot be won by natural means. Their roots go deeper to an invisible place with unseen forces that do their best work through our ignorance. After all other efforts have failed, it's time to look deeper and let God show us the root of the fruit that is showing up in our lives, on our hips, and on our lips. Sometimes we have to get past ourselves to see what's really in the way. The truth hurts, but it's also medicine that can set you free. So don't despise the process. Hang in there, my sister.

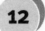

12

Extreme Makeovers

I THOUGHT MY WEIGHT ISSUES were all about how cute I felt I was or wasn't, but little did I know that things were about to get a whole lot deeper than my surface concerns. After I ran into a looking-too-fabulous-for-words friend of mine in LA, she revealed her secret was Dr. Keith Richardson, an iridologist who had changed her life. I made an appointment right away. So there I sat with Dr. Richardson looking into my eyes through the lens of a machine that magnified all of my sins. . . . I felt like the woman at the well.[1] You know—the story where Jesus read all her personal mail in one conversation. He told her all about herself, and they had never met before. She was flabbergasted. Can you imagine a stranger just walking up to you and telling you all your personal business? The embarrassing stuff you don't want anyone to know? Uh-huh, that's what Dr. Richardson was doing. He would look through the lens of his little machine and then go, "Mmm. . . ." Then he would write copious notes on his notepad and then lean forward to peer into my eyes again. This went on for about a half hour. To tell you the truth, I was getting worried. Finally he looked up long enough for me to ask, "Is it really that bad?"

"Only if you want to live," he replied.

With that, he looked down at his paper and began telling me all my business: the number of surgeries I'd had, the number of fibroids in my body and exactly where they were. When he mentioned the fibroids, my jaw dropped; it hit the table when he told me about the lumps I had in my breast. I had just had an ultrasound and mammogram the week before and been told about them. He then went on to tell me my stress level was through the ceiling and I had to do something about my life! Whew—all of that from just looking into my eyes! My iridologist then proceeded to ban me from eating chicken. Chicken, Dr. Richardson said, was chock-full of hormones that just exacerbated my female issues. He told me that the hormones in meat that was not farm fed and organic simply fed my system more hormones that just added fuel to the fire already raging in my body.

An hour later, I left Dr. Richardson's office, armed with a shopping bag filled with about eight bottles of different types of herbal tablets designed to cleanse different parts of my body from my glands to my urine, a twelve-ounce bottle of virgin olive oil, and a sheet of instructions for a twenty-one-day program of cleansing my system. I was off to restore my body to perfect health.

"Remember, no chicken!" he said before acknowledging another lady who slipped in the door I had just exited. "Yes, sir!" I said before heading to El Pollo Loco to have one last wing-lovers special before dedicating my body to cleansing.

Well, I must tell you that only the strong survive the first day of this program. After taking a mild mixture of herbs called Colontone that acted as a laxative for three nights to prepare myself for the cleanse, the "first" day of this program officially arrived. I was told to mix eight ounces of olive oil with lemon juice and drink the whole concoction. The very next instruction was, "Don't lie down." But the mixture of all that oil and lemon juice made me nauseated, so I lay down to settle my stomach. In no time flat, the fun began. I dashed for the bathroom, not knowing if I should sit or stand as both my stomach and my colon threatened to erupt at the same time. The contents were trying to escape through any opening they could find. I'm not trying to be gross or anything, but this was the most violent cleanse I had ever experienced. The olive oil literally coated the walls of my colon and made everything that tried to cling to my intestinal walls slide out. I had an image of the last dregs of old food trying to hang on to anything they could to secure their place in my system but to no avail. Nothing was safe. It was frightening. Who knew the body could harbor so much horrible stuff?! Talk about bubble, bubble, toil, and trouble! Needless to say, my commode and I became inseparable friends until finally, at the end of the day, my body heaved a great sigh of relief and returned to normalcy. Finally, everything and everyone was out.

I didn't even think about food. If I had, I doubt I would have been able to eat it. I was now haunted by the memory of what food turned into. The next day, I began the regimen of taking five of each of the other herbs I had been given every two hours. I was surprised that I was not hungry and had energy to burn. In fact, I felt downright good! After seven days, I was able to add fruit and vegetables; the last seven days, I added grains; and the last four days, I was able to add fish. I went down two dress sizes, and for the first time in my life, my stomach was flat! I felt great. My skin glowed. I looked hot! I ran and bought a cute, body-skimming black dress and took pictures. The results were so drastic that I decided to obey Dr. Richardson and continue not to eat chicken. Three months later, I was still slim and trim and a lot healthier than I knew. I returned for another checkup to find that my fibroids had shrunk and the lumps in my breast were gone!

My insides felt so nice and clean that I didn't want to sully them with anything that would clog them up ever again. My publicist encouraged me to write about how I had lost all my weight for magazines, but I was too busy shopping! And traveling.

Aye! And that is where I met my demise this time . . . on the road. It was subtle, and once again, one cheat led to another and another. A sad thing happens when you get too tired or allow yourself to get too hungry before you eat. You eat all the wrong things. I decided to do whatever I had to do to catch myself before things got too out of hand. So in order to recover what I had lost, my trainer (I called him "Mr. Fine," though his real name was Victor) suggested I do the bodybuilder trick for losing weight and build muscle instead of fat. It was a simple and boring regimen. In the morning I had egg whites and some vegetables or some oatmeal, and every three hours or so I had about three ounces of lean protein and some vegetables. No carbs (as in bread, rice, you know what I'm talking about—all the stuff we love). Lots of water and cardio. Ah yes, that would be exercise—as in thirty minutes to an hour on a bike or a treadmill. Cardio meant doing something that made you sweat and burn fat. Exercise . . . what a novel concept, but we'll talk about that later.

This down and dirty recipe for getting lean and mean worked, too. I saw my jawline come back, and my arms even had little cuts in them. I was bordering on buff, but the boredom of the same old stuff to eat over and over, and having to remember to eat every couple of hours, pushed me over the edge, and you guessed it— back into the arms of a fried chicken wing. It was all over but the shouting and wails of regret after that.

One good slip deserves another and another and another until you lose track and give up altogether. My fat was happy to see me. The reunion with my old clothing made me sad, but as I told you before, I clean up very well, so I just went back to my former duds and pretended that nothing had happened. I think they tried to chastise me for straying. Dr. Richardson called to check on my progress several times, but like a guilty lover gone astray, I avoided him.

The moral of the story? Extremes may work (and work well), but they lessen your willpower for sticking with a permanent way of eating that will maintain your losses. My mind and my heart still had not made the shift to where I needed to be attitudinally; therefore, every diet was an unfaithful lover leaving me in worse shape after a brief dalliance. Ah, but it was fun while it lasted.

Still, the question remained: When would I have a lasting affair? So much for the journey of getting to the end of myself. I still wasn't there. But the pendulum was swinging a little closer to the center than when I'd started, and that was encouraging. At least I knew my sins when it came to food, and I had learned that I had the power to achieve my goal if I really wanted to. But balancing what I knew with consistent action was the key. That much I knew. I assured myself I was on my way to finding balance one way or the other.

KEEPING IT REAL

- Make a list of all the extreme measures you've taken to lose weight.

- What was the outcome of these eating experiences?

- How much weight did you gain back?

- What was your reaction to the weight gain? What made it hard for you to put the brakes on what you were eating?

- What are the eating traps in your life? How can you avoid them? What things can you put in place to give you support and keep you on track?

- What balance do you need to find in your eating?

DIVA REFLECTIONS

You will be consumed by whatever you focus on. That is fact. The fight to get food off my mind has been one of my greatest struggles. It's true. Food is a drug. It releases things in our systems that compensate for every other emotion we experience. When we go to extremes, we can only press past the things that brought us to this place temporarily. Like a boomerang, we bounce back to the place we abandoned too quickly to carve a new path for our desires. The good part is that, somewhere between the opposites of going to the extreme, is a beautiful place called balance that we can all reach if we refuse to give up.

Who Ya Gonna Call?

"HAVE YOU CALLED JENNY YET?" Kirstie Alley happily chirped as she pranced across the screen. I wanted to reach into the TV and slap her. She had invited the nation to watch her lose weight, and we all cheered her on. I'm sure half of the group were waiting like vultures circling fresh meat to see how long it would take her to fall off the horse. Well, as you know, she eventually did, shortly after modeling a swimsuit on Oprah. (I knew that was the kiss of death right there.) Something happens when we finally hit that goal and get too confident. And we could all empathize with her because we had been there too. But the weight loss crusade continued on with other stars such as Valerie Bertinelli, who lived to write a book about it, and Queen Latifah, who was smart enough not to have unrealistic expectations and focus on her health (I love that girl!).

Now don't call me a hater, 'cause I'm not. As you know by now, based on some of my previous admissions, all my fellow diva dieters finally sucked me into trying their diets. I, too, could proudly chirp, "I called Jenny! She's my new BFF!" But I've made the rounds and also called Nutrisystem, Diet Center, Weight Watchers, and last, but not least, my newest discovery, Seattle Sutton.

Here is my blanket review of them all. Humor me as I put on my Roger Ebert hat for diets. Picture me seated on a beautiful chaise, dressed in black, of course, hair flowing, noshing casually on popcorn while I serve up my discourse on all the various weight-management programs as if they were a hit movie.

It's hard to label *The Amazing Shrinking Woman*. At various points, what seems to be a comedy makes the sharp turn to a drama when the plot thickens along with the heroine's waistline. The supporting cast of those who encourage her are juxtaposed against a bevy of antagonists who seem to delight in thwarting the attempts of the heroine to stay on course with her mission to lose weight; these antagonists heap false praise on her when she is most vulnerable, and they offer her the things they know are her weakness (like chocolate cake!). The opening scene paints a picture of deep introspection as our heroine faces the truth about herself and makes the decision that she needs help. But who does she get help from? Well-meaning friends who agree to do a group diet contest? Does she sign on with Dr. Ian's countrywide 50 Million Pound Challenge or his 4 Day Diet? Does she submit to the cherubic encouragement of Richard Simmons? Or sign up for an experimental liquid diet at a hospital, do the Medifast, seek hands-on accountability with a weight-management program? Her struggles are riveting as she tries one, then the other—having some measure of success with each until she can't bear to continue. In one scene, where she admits food is her drug, her pain is palpable. She takes the viewers on a drastic pendulum swing of emotions as her weight rises and falls along with her self-esteem and her romantic options. She is a sympathetic character we can all relate to as we compare our own struggles with hers. I'm sure there will be a sequel to this hilarious yet real-life adventure because, based on the many fluctuations the heroine experienced, I'm sure she will be trying many more "diets" with equally interesting scenarios. After all, if she just chose to make peace with her body, there would be no more drama, would there? The end, by the diva of dietary critique—that would be me—Michelle McKinney Hammond, signing off to get a snack.

Lets' face it: When it comes to diet plans, there are sooo many options and sooo many ways to take off the weight, there could be various reality sitcoms that feature stars (and everyday folks like you and me) struggling to lose weight season after season. What? You say you already did that? Uh-huh, the struggle with weight is totally not an original concept. So perhaps that's where you should start when you are ready to take off the weight for good. Take a deep breath and say to yourself, "I am not alone." All right. That being said, let's make a realistic evaluation to see if you need help from one of these programs or not. Why do you think you need help? And what kind of help do you need? (There's emotional support, help choosing foods, a trainer to help with exercise, etc.) If you are severely overweight, you may need to consult with a physician on this one.

I want to make one simple request that we just agree to stop the yo-yo effect. It's time to get focused, get serious, and covenant with ourselves to walk in agreement that we are all going to do this one step at a time. Be patient with yourself. It didn't take you one day to gain all that weight, and it's not going to take you one day (or one week or even one month) to lose it. Now that we have that out of the way, you have to take stock of your lifestyle and habits to determine what you need to do about those hips, girlfriend.

Everybody I know screwed up their faces when Lady O (that

would be Oprah) lost her weight (the last time). They all said, "If I had her money and could hire my own chef, I'd lose weight too!" So what's your excuse? You can hire your own chef too. Her name is Jenny. Jenny Craig. Or you can call Nutri. As in Nutrisystem. Or you can just skip the whole thing and do the Medifast! There's more than one way to skin the fat off your thighs, sister girl. Ah, but here's the rub (no pun intended): None of these programs were designed to be permanent ways of eating. If you continued eating prepackaged food, your system would blow up from sodium overload. If you only had protein shakes, soup, and oatmeal, you'd look like a rather sad prune after a while, and you would be rather evil, too. After a while everything would look good. You would find yourself chomping on someone's dried-flower arrangement. Even hiring your own cook can be a temporary fix; what happens when you travel? Or are invited out to eat? Or you can't afford your cook anymore? Or your cook goes on to have his own show?

What you must understand before you get started with all or any of these diets or plans is that the programs are there to *reprogram you* until you can stand on your own two feet. Most of the time, the biggest hurdle with anyone who has a weight problem is portion control. It's not always what you eat; it's how much and when you eat that creates the most problems. For the most part, I have always been guilty of not eating enough. Now, that worked when I was young, but when my metabolism changed, it created problems. I would literally forget to eat all day and then make up for it with one huge meal after seven o'clock. Then while I slept on it, my hips and stomach stored everything I ate before I went to bed. Get the picture? I see you nodding your head. We can't do that anymore. Repeat after me: no, no, no, no can do anymore. Sing it if you have to. So let's look for common threads of agreement here with all the diet programs. They all tell you the key is eating small portions often. You should be putting something beneficial in your mouth five to six times a day. You've got to get that engine burning. Wake up that body, and make it do the work it's supposed to do. That's right. Tell your metabolism the vacation is over!

So if you don't want to eat three weeks free after paying for the first several weeks with one program or don't have money for the sign-up fee with another, you can do this at home if you really want to, but it's going to take some planning on your part. Here's my suggestion: Plan your work, then work your plan.

First we begin with the menu. Choose low maintenance—low- to no-prep items that are still delicious. Cut up all your vegetables, put your salads in containers to make meal-sized portions for the week, cook your meats, prepare your toppings. You get where this is going? That's right! You can have your meals ready ahead of time and heat them up just as if you had bought them. You can pick up a couple of Lean Cuisines to supplement your homemade dishes and have your own program for less money! However, I won't be mad at you if you need to get on a roll by submitting yourself to one of the prearranged diet plans first. Whatever works is what you have to do.

My suggestion is that you join a weight-management program and do it until your stomach shrinks, you drop enough weight to feel committed to continuing to do the right thing by your body, and you begin to get used to the smaller portions. Then hold that thought and begin to prepare your meals yourself, using the same portions. This is how you make the transition from a supervised diet to a lifestyle change.

If we were really honest, most of us don't cook anymore, and that creates a major problem because we go for a long time until we get hungry. Then as we stand before the empty refrigerator, we run out and buy something that is bad for us and eat the whole thing—no matter how much food it is. (Just raise your hand and say, "Guilty.") So what are you going to do about that, huh? You are going to have to either learn how to cook or call "Joe," as in Trader Joe's, or Whole Foods. These two stores are a haven for pre-cooked meals that you can heat up and watch your weight at the same time. My favorite from Trader Joe's is the Korean short ribs; you heat them up two minutes on each side and slap them next to a salad, and you are transported to the south side of heaven. Yummy! Don't stop there. Go on down the aisle, pick up some crab-stuffed salmon or some seasoned chicken breasts. If you can't cook (or don't want to cook), there are plenty of people cooking for you. Why do I suggest these two stores in particular? Because they are dedicated to three terms that are important on your dietary journey: *low sodium*, *natural*, and *organic*. (If you look hard enough, you may be able to find natural and organic foods in other grocery stores as well, but remember to read the labels!) The last thing you need when you're trying to lose pounds is stuff loaded down with a ton of preservatives, sodium, sugar, or hormones. Let's think about this a minute. Sodium makes you retain water, and hormones make stuff bigger. If you eat something that is pumped up with hormones, what do you think it's going to do to you? I thought you would see my point. The bottom line of this entire conversation? If you can't cook, there is help for you. If you don't have money to call Jenny or a weight-management program that charges a fee, don't use that as an excuse for not trying.

Last, but certainly not least, get an accountability partner. My sister and I agreed to hold one another accountable. We didn't have to reveal our weight to one another, God forbid, but daily we had to e-mail or call one another with the full list of what we had eaten for the day and what exercise we had done. A huge part of staying on track is the knowledge that you will have to face someone with your failures and have a partner to celebrate your victories. As long as you remain honest with yourselves and one another, you will see results. So make a pact with friends, family, or coworkers. (Or you can start your own club.) Where there's a will, there's a way; so don't just sit there getting wider—call somebody!

KEEPING IT REAL

- To the best of your memory, what is the common thread to all the diets you've done before? What worked for you? What didn't work for you? Consider the results. How much did you gain back afterward?

- Write a resolution that goes something like this: "Today is the end of my dieting cycle. From this day forth, I will be the master of my body and my diet. I will be wise. I will be consistent. I will embrace a new attitude toward eating that will agree with my heart and my body. I will be victorious!"

- Choose a weight-management program or an accountability partner who is appropriate for your needs.

- Make a list of your favorite foods. Find the healthy things that will be beneficial to your new mode of eating, and stock up.

- Plan your menu, and go forth and conquer!

- Write down everything that goes into your mouth. There is something about the facts staring at you from a piece of paper that will keep you sober, or at least kick you back on track if you veer off on a tangent.

DIVA REFLECTIONS

No one ever said being the boss of your body would be easy, but that doesn't mean it's impossible. Being realistic about your weaknesses is the beginning to gaining victory. Pride and shame will try to make you do it alone, but isolation is the greatest factor of any failure. Community is about more than sharing things. It's about lending strength and well-placed guidance to one another. That is when the journey becomes a joyful one, no matter how difficult. Sometimes just knowing you're not alone is enough to help you over the finish line.

14

Eenie, Meenie, Minie, Yo-Yo!

AS I RUMMAGED through my closet, mourning over all the things I could no longer squeeze into, and moved all my larger outfits and things with elastic to the front for easier access, I considered joining my friend Jeff on yet another extreme makeover—à la the Atkins Diet. Yeah, you know the one where you consume massive quantities of protein. Eggs, bacon, cheese—lots of protein and fat. No vegetables. No juice. No fruit. No dairy. No carbs. Wait a minute. No fruit? That did it for me. I decided any diet that tells you to forsake the natural stuff God created and recommended you eat in the Bible—as in seedbearing plants (that would be fruits and vegetables)—couldn't be on track.[1] Plus, eating all that meat and fat on the Atkins Diet sounded like a heart attack waiting to happen to me. I just decided all that stuff with nothing sweet to wash it down had to contribute to backing up your arteries. I must say that my friend Jeff lost a lot of weight on this diet. He diligently stuck to it and was lean and mean in no time. But the island girl in me just couldn't get past the no-fruit mandate. And of course, eventually Jeff couldn't continue his protein course and gained the weight back.

By now I had concluded that dieting was like a relationship. You know how it is. During the first flush of attraction, you are all excited; to woo the person, you do things you know you can't keep up. After you feel secure that you've locked the person and relationship in, you relax, get comfortable, and let all the romantic gestures and extra stuff you were doing begin to fall by the wayside. This causes problems. The neglected partner begins to wonder what is wrong. You might hear, "Don't you love me anymore?" The decline of your earlier extras has an impact on the relationship, and not for the good. This could be the beginning of the end if you don't go back to doing what you did to get your mate in the first place. What it took to get that person into your life is the same thing it will take to keep that person. After all, that is why your mate fell in love with you in the first place. Yes, the long and short of it is that you should never start habits you can't maintain or do anything that is not natural for you; you won't be able to keep it up. This always causes problems that can lead to the demise of what you desired. Upon that realization and correlation between dating and losing weight, I decided to try to find a more balanced approach to weight loss that allowed me to eat not only things of the seed-bearing persuasion but all the rest of the things I knew I liked to eat.

About the time of my balanced realization, my parents had embarked on the South Beach Diet. The results were amazing. My parents looked like newlyweds. Not only were they svelte, but they also gained some health benefits as a result of their new eating habits. In fact, one day after they had been on the diet for a while, my dad, a diabetic, passed out and was rushed to the hospital only to find that his blood sugar level had gone back to normal levels. He no longer needed insulin! Not only was he now a slim goody, but he was good and healthy.

When my parents came to visit me, they came bearing a cooler with all their supplies to fix their meals. Ah, yes, with balance came work. There were meals to prepare and snacks to be had at regular intervals throughout the day. My mother was now consumed with cooking most of the day. After breakfast, it was time to get lunch prepared, and then dinner; she was busy preparing three meals and two snacks a day. But this became their ritual that they truly enjoyed.

The South Beach Diet is progressive. During the initial phase, you cut out carbs, but you add them back in as the diet progresses. This diet is about learning how to eat all things in balance. There are all sorts of delightful recipes and wonderful concoctions cooked the low-fat way that give you the enjoyment of eating all the things you love with the added bonus of eating your way to slimness. This diet was a delight for my two retired parents, who loved to cook. I was happy for them. They had the time. I, on the other hand, did not. And that's key to finding what works for you: knowing what you can do and knowing what you can't do. I could not cook three meals and two snacks a day.

What's a busy career girl to do? Call Jenny! That's right. I called Jenny Craig. I marched right down to one of her diet facilities, stood on that scale, and subjected myself to someone recording the number I didn't want to face. Then they sat me down with a list of all their meals and let me pick what I wanted! All kinds of yummy concoctions. And the snacks. Wow! The Cheese Curls were my favorite. But the meals were delicious and easy to keep up with in my daily regimen and hectic schedule. All I had to do was slap those bad puppies in the microwave, and any given meal was ready in minutes. Add some salad, and you were on your way to skinny. And I was . . . until I traveled. Now mind you, I was determined to eat Jenny's food. I had lost eight pounds in four weeks and had hope for the future. Nothing was going to stand between me and my new, skinny self, not even an ocean. So I packed up my suitcase with all my food and dragged it all the way to London, where the best-laid plans of mice and men crumbled quickly.

The dear friend I was visiting had taken it upon herself to hire a cook to prepare all manner of delicacies for me for the duration of my entire trip! Eddie, the cook I decided I must kidnap the moment I became rich and famous, was a master in the kitchen; however, he laughed in the face of the word *diet* while waving all manner of specialty dishes under my nose. My resolve crumbled, making me an unfaithful lover once again. Jenny was going to have to wait until I got back home. In the face of Eddie's creamy French sauces and other rich food, Jenny's prepackaged fare didn't stand a chance. As I closed my eyes and chewed, savoring all the flavors dancing on my tongue, I decided the pounds I would gain back during this trip would be worth it.

But there is nothing like dieter's remorse to make you hate yourself—that's for sure. A week later after schlepping all my Jenny meals back across the ocean in my suitcase, it took a moment to warm back up to my little prepackaged meals. Thoughts of Eddie's beignets kept dancing through my head as I tried to focus on my string beans. I resolved that I would not be taking Jenny to Africa later in the year. As I started to watch my travel calendar fill up, I knew that Jenny could not be my BFF for long. I was gone too much for us to have the type of relationship we needed to have for this diet to work.

So how was I going to be able to travel and watch my weight? Weight Watchers! About this time, my friend Terri proudly proclaimed she had reached her goal weight and had lost forty pounds in one year. She looked great. I was jealous. And still fat. I was still bouncing up and down between the same five pounds I had been trying to lose for forever. Terri encouraged me to just get started. She would coach me. I wasn't interested in counting points, so I chose the simple formula of five fruits and vegetables, two servings of three ounces of lean protein, two servings of dairy, and eight glasses of water per day. Three meals, two snacks, simple and sweet. This left me with thirty-five points that I could use for extra stuff. Since I'm not a big dessert person, I kept the extra points for the condiments I can't do without—ketchup, salad dressing, etc.

I have to tell you, this was working for me! It was easy for me to do the math. I concocted a way to stay on top of what I had to eat. I made up my little menu for the week, and off to the grocery store I went. I cooked up my chicken breast. Gathered cans of tuna. Cut up my vegetables for a week's worth of salad. Chopped up my fruits to make a delicious fruit salad I could have in between eating whole pieces of fruit. I was in heaven. I supplemented my water with hot herbal teas and bottles of smart water swirling with Crystal Light, and I was doing great! This was something I could keep up when I traveled simply by making the right choices when ordering food. I didn't feel deprived because my cheats just had to stay within the realm of my thirty-five points, which I plotted and planned out with passion.

I was steadily losing the weight—not by leaps and bounds, but on a consistent basis. I also felt so much better. My system seemed to thank me as it embraced a cleaner diet. I had decided quite some time ago that simple carbs were not my friends. So my passionate love affair with bread ended, unless it was a piece worth cheating for. Baked potatoes were relegated to a once-a-month treat, while rice was limited to half a cup every full moon. Sacrifices had to be made in the name of vanity if this was going to work.

I can't say when or where I slipped off the wagon this time, but I did. I say slipped because there was no marked fall. Perhaps it was around my birthday when I gave in to eating every cupcake in the box that someone so lovingly bought for me. (Don't you just love it when your friends love you to death by giving you all manner of sweets that you have no business eating?) Or maybe it was the holiday barbeque where I loaded up on mounds of creamy potato salad (it was so good I tried to inhale the whole bowl); I really can't say where I went wrong. But the pounds I had been losing first screeched to a frustratingly dead halt, and then they switched into reverse. My girlfriend Terri asked me if I had been exercising. I don't think I answered the question, but the sting of it made me avoid talking to her for a few days. She got the hint. We never spoke of it again.

Now that I was officially not watching my weight anymore because the scale depressed me too much, I went back to my old ways of eating whatever, whenever I wanted with no good results, but I pretended not to care until I couldn't stand myself any longer. As I sat pondering what to do with myself next, I took stock of my past failures and looked for keys to what had made my best-laid plans fail so miserably.

First, I realized I was totally undisciplined. I couldn't keep up with all the times I was supposed to eat. I forgot to eat in the midst of my busy day and usually crumbled into a ravenous heap by the end of the day, craving everything that was loaded with fat to fill me up quickly. By then, I didn't want anything that was good for me, only things that fooled me into thinking I felt good. Yummy, creamy, saucy things—the kind that stuck to my ribs and made my taste buds feel alive. And gave me gas later. (Let's be real here.)

Food preparation was also a problem for me. I just did not have time. This was my downfall. When I had time to preprepare everything, I did well; when I didn't, which was more often than not, I floundered and sank.

Food portions were also a biggie, no pun intended. By the time I got around to eating, not only did I reach for the wrong things, but I consumed too much of them. All of these things needed to be brought into balance. And while Jenny had done a great job of bringing all these things into submission through her prepackaged meals, I couldn't go back to her. The one issue I had with all the prepackaged meals was the high level of sodium. There were days when my body was slimmer but my ankles were not.

Enter stage right: Seattle Sutton. It was like having my own personal chef! Healthy and fresh (not frozen) meals were delivered to my door every Monday and Thursday for a fraction of what I had been spending on groceries myself! I felt like Oprah, except I couldn't see who was cooking my food. The meals were portioned to the right calorie count for me. Breakfast, lunch, dinner, snack, salad, fruit—everything was included except my serving of dairy. The price was right, the food was delicious, and once again, I was on my way back toward the size ten Michael Kors suit I refused to part with. When I traveled, I simply told the folks at Seattle Sutton not to deliver food until I got back. All was well until my phone started ringing with various and sundry invites to eat out. I never realized how much I ate out until I looked at my Seattle leftovers piling up and spoiling in my refrigerator. It exposed my lack of discipline. *Why do I say yes when I need to say no?* I asked myself. Ironically, I had written a book on the subject but hadn't followed my own advice. It wasn't as if the world and all those restaurants wouldn't still be there by the time I got a handle on my weight. Well . . . perhaps they wouldn't be. Still, I persisted in patronizing them, chiefly because I liked the food and the convenience of not having to deal with cooking. So after several international trips back-to-back and my continuing to enjoy dining out when home, Seattle and I were destined to have a long-distance relationship. However, after breaking up with Seattle, I noticed something. I had not gained back what I had lost. As I pondered this miracle, I noticed something else. The way I ate had changed. I ate smaller portions! Had my stomach shrunk, or had something finally connected with the discipline that Jenny, Weight Watchers, and Seattle had been trying to instill in me? I think it was a combination of both. To be honest, I really didn't care. I was just relieved to feel that I was finally getting somewhere. It's amazing what happens when you feel that way. New hope rises and gives you the strength to begin to do the right thing—and that, my friend, is the goal.

KEEPING IT REAL

- Write a list of the things that keep you from eating the way you should.

- What types of pressures are you under timewise? What stops you from eating regularly throughout the day?

- What steps can you take to begin to make sure you eat at regular intervals?

- Examine your portions. What do you need to cut back on? Be honest about why you eat as much as you do.

- Determine which program would be best for you to help you get disciplined in your approach to eating.

- Get rid of the weight gain section in your closet—you know, all the big and expandable stuff. (Raise your hand with me if you're guilty. These are props that support your yo-yo syndrome.) Needing new clothes can be an expensive consequence to a diet out of control. Perhaps if you can't get in the clothes you have, you will be motivated to stop your weight gain earlier because it will cost you something.

DIVA REFLECTIONS

Somewhere between eating too much and eating too little is a beautiful place called "just enough." Just enough for what? For being full, satisfied, healthy, and guilt free. Once again, when the war between your body and your taste buds has been settled, your body will have a fighting chance to be true to itself, giving you the freedom to make the right choices for both of you. I believe the body tells us what it wants, but it gets confused when we don't treat it properly. You must be the parent and make the right choices until your palate and your stomach are reeducated. Trust me, your body will not only begin to line up; it will thank you for it in the long run.

15

What's Really Eating You?

YOU GUESSED IT—I fell off the horse again. That's right. After all that romance with Jenny Craig, Weight Watchers, Seattle Sutton, and my own newly designed portion controls, somehow my stomach expanded and I was happy to once again accommodate all its yearnings. I had to get to the bottom of why this happened once and for all, for my health's sake as well as for yours.

I am fascinated by people who lose weight when they are in distress. I am not among that number. I recall when my friend Annette was having trouble at her job, she dropped twenty pounds just like that. (I think I found her lost pounds, but that's beside the point.) She said that she "just forgot to eat" and was so stressed out and worried that she involuntarily turned into the gaunt woman who now stood before me. I preferred to blame it on the streets of New York and the subway systems with escalators that never worked. *If I lived in New York and couldn't catch a cab, I'd be skinny too*, I rationalized. Then, there was my girlfriend Cindy, who tragically lost her husband. Again, she, too, turned into a cuter version of Twiggy. I scratched my head. The opposite occurred when I was in distress or stressed. I became an incessant nibbler, *and* I ate full meals that had lots of cream and carbs. There is a reason they call this stuff "comfort food." I am here to tell you that on a day when I have been pushed past the limit and over the edge, potatoes and some gravy with mushrooms swimming in it is like drugs to me. The first bite has the same effect on me that I've seen drug addicts have in the movies after they take a hit. It is followed by a huge sigh of gratitude and a settling into bliss. Depending on how long my crisis or angst lasted, I was sure to consume massive quantities of macaroni and cheese, Stouffer's Spinach Soufflé, followed by their sautéed Harvest Apples, followed by Brie and marmalade baked in a pastry . . . can you see where this is going besides my waistline? Uh-huh, I thought you knew!

My mental panic did not help as I realized what I was doing to myself. It was as if I had gotten on a roller-coaster ride, and the operator had vacated his post, leaving me screaming as the car descended downward at breakneck speed. How to get off the ride while it careened out of control was not a present option, or so it seemed. It was at this point that I realized something had to be done.

My life is highly stressful. No ifs, ands, or buts about it. Well . . . if my butt was any indication, I might have to take that statement back. But anyhow, back to the point—take a deep breath and repeat after me: *It is not what I put* into *my mouth, but rather what comes* out *of it that can cause me more damage than I know.* I know what you are thinking—that sounds backward. But trust me, it's not. I realized that the more I nursed and rehearsed all the dramas and demands in my life out loud, the more I would get myself really worked up, and the only thing that distracted me from full-blown hysteria was eating, because it made me shut up temporarily.

I think it was one of those Relacore commercials that turned on the light for me. As the little diagram of a woman's tubby middle circled on-screen, the announcer went on and on about how stress can pile on the pounds at our centers. Stress, the announcer said, released some hormone called cortisol that helped fat cells replicate and herd around our middles, where they not only ruin the lines of that favorite little black dress, but also pose a dangerous threat to the heart. Basically, stress contributes to fat's crowding vital organs and lining the arteries with fatty stuff that could turn to plaque and slow down blood flow to the heart—and that is more serious than just the tubby middle stress can create. That's when I got the first clue of what had been happening to me. I knew it would take more than a pill to correct my situation. It was time to master my emotions and not give in to eating every time a situation had me "eyebrows to scalp" in my life, making me look more crazy than dismayed.

For most of us, unlike my friends Annette and Cindy, stress doesn't make us drop pounds. It makes us eat more. In our stressful states, our bodies can't break down food as they should because we've distracted the energy elsewhere. The body is interesting. When we eat, the system goes to work breaking down the food, assimilating the nutrients into the bloodstream, and discarding the wastes. Our blood is actively involved in this, which is perhaps why when we eat too much, we feel lightheaded or sleepy—'cause all the blood has left the building (your brain), so to speak, to try and break down all this food and keep it moving. Our blood is very busy. All the blood in our systems dashes to wherever there is a hurt in order to do the work of repairing the malady. So let's add stress to this mix, which gets the system off kilter. Then you add more food and more fat, and your body has to work extra hard; eventually, it can't keep up with your eating, and it leaves the fat from those leftovers around your middle, which is not good for your heart—emotionally or physically. It is also believed that midsection fat—besides being bad for your heart—usually indicates other stuff, like cholesterol, is collecting in your system. (This is just bad news all around—once again, no pun intended!)

In the movie *What's Eating Gilbert Grape*, Gilbert's mother was huge; her weight didn't just affect her; it affected her entire family and put undue stress on her children. Your weight will never just affect your body. It will affect your mental state. How you respond to the situations in your life. Your relationships. Your work. Your everything. You can't afford to be out of control, because it can have a negative effect on too many things. Yet, the very things that are important to us—our relationships, our work—can work against us and make us self-destruct without realizing it.

There are lots of things that can eat away at us and drive us to the worst solution—eating. Perhaps it all began the day your mother gave you a cookie when you cried after falling and skinning your knee. You learned early that food could distract you from your pain. The part we missed was that sometimes food (or using food to medicate) could also cause us more suffering.

Then there is the absentminded nibbling that can come from stress, nervousness, and worry. This occurs when you don't even realize that you're mindlessly snacking until the entire bag of potato chips is empty or the whole pint of ice cream is gone . . . can I get a witness? What is the answer to this incessant craving to make ourselves feel better? The answer is far from obvious. I'm sure you could come up with practical stuff like locking all your cabinets that have anything sweet in them, or avoiding any place that might harbor fattening things you like, or torturing yourself by putting your mouth on lockdown while your mind drives you crazy with visions of chocolate and other soothing confections. Or you can go inward and deal with what is really going on with you.

Have you ever gotten up in the middle of the night, craving God only knows what? You go to the refrigerator and you look in, but nothing is calling your name. Yet you are hungry, starving (or so you think). So you open up a container of whatever leftovers are there. You taste it. It's not quite what your taste buds crave, but you eat it anyway. Well, about three containers later, you're stuffed but still not satisfied. Perhaps it was not your body that was hungry.

I can testify to this from my own experience. When I am fasting instead of eating a meal, I read my Bible, and my hunger goes away. I believe that most of the time when we are hungry outside of mealtime, our spirit is really the driving force of our hunger. No food—well, no food of the mashed-potato-and-meat variety—will ever satisfy our souls, and perhaps this is why we don't feel satisfied when we raid the fridge. Let's face it: There is a difference between being full and being satisfied. In the midst of our stress and anxiety, the spirit's hunger is amplified because it knows that we were not designed to carry around our fears, need for love and security, or concerns. We are supposed to give them to God because He cares for us and holds the answers we are struggling to find.[1] The more we wrestle within ourselves, the greater our hunger becomes. But when we unload our worries in prayer and/ or seek additional counseling if need be, we release the things that are driving us to make physically detrimental choices. Slowing down the beating of our racing hearts allows the blood to go back to our brains where it belongs and feed it with the strength we need to gain clarity. As I silence my thoughts and determine to be still and know that He is God, He is magnified, becoming bigger than all my problems and needs.[2] Things come into perspective as they should, and I am able to release the things that threatened to make me careen out of control.

Releasing is huge for a control freak like me. It is not in my nature to let go of things. I wrestle things to the floor, not realizing most of the time that I'm the one pressed against the mat. Ah, but when I release my cares to God, suddenly the only thing I'm left wrestling is myself and my own tendencies to choose the path of least resistance—like a snack! And that's why I don't turn to prayer in those moments as often as I should. Then there is no excuse for me to feed my face, and I would rather cling to my pain and the food that does not satisfy or nourish me.

Recently I was watching a love story with Emma Thompson and Dustin Hoffman. Dustin was determined to win Emma's heart in spite of her resistance. Her character said the most profound thing. She said to Dustin, "Perhaps I am more comfortable living with disappointment, and I am angry at you for taking that away from me." That's it. It's too difficult to give things to God because it leaves me with no acceptable reason for doing the things I do. Or maybe it is my ego at work. My ego doesn't like the idea that there is someone bigger or greater than myself. It doesn't like to confess that sometimes the issues I wrestle with are bigger than me. I like thinking I'm lord of my life and personal universe, and yet the truth of the matter is, I am not. Neither are you. But we all have this false obligation to solve all our dramas. No matter how much I know intellectually that God will always allow things to creep into my world that magnify my need for Him, I keep duking it out with my problems until I crumble in an exhausted heap, crawling back to the foot of the cross. Finally, I'm willing to open my bloody little hands and release my fears, my questions, and my problems. In that moment, I wonder why I held on and fought so long. Yes, it is pride mingled with fear and uncertainty of what would happen if I really let go. And yet there is something inside of us all that is secretly relieved when we open our hands and stop clinging to things we can't solve. The sigh of relief can be exaggerated. Just don't pick up a fork in the next breath!

Of course, physical activity (that would be exercise) is a great stress buster. All those racing thoughts and energy have to go somewhere . . . but more on this in a later chapter. For now, be willing to step in front of the mirror and look yourself in the eye and be honest with yourself. Don't look in the mirror and then walk away, forgetting what you saw. That is the worst self-deception of all. Make an honest assessment of your emotional and psychological state. Speak the truth and not a lie: "Girlfriend, you are stressed out!" Now open your palms and repeat after me: "I am going to release this issue to God until I get further marching orders from Him, 'cause I can't do anything about something I can do nothing about." Make sense? You may not be able to do anything, but God can. However, He does hold you responsible for mastering your emotions and making wise choices. So release what you need to release in order for Him to do His part, and stick to doing what you can do. Now, take a deep breath, count to ten, relax, and release all that upper-body tension along with your issue, take a walk, and grab a carrot stick (if you need something to eat).

KEEPING IT REAL

- Make a list of your top-five stress factors.

- Evaluate if there is anything you can do about these situations. For those that you can, write three things you need to do to correct the issue. For those you cannot, put those in a separate list labeled "Prayer Concerns." Write a statement of release for these things.

- Seek counseling from a wise source who is successful in the area you are struggling with.

- Find a physical activity that will help you release pent-up anxiety and refocus your thoughts.

- Shake off false guilt about not tackling every situation. Accept your humanity in light of God's power to deal with the impossibilities in your life.

- Get a good eight hours of sleep. Sleep is not only a time when the body mends itself and de-stresses, but a good night's sleep can also help you lose weight.

DIVA REFLECTIONS

I've discovered that the more I nurse and rehearse a situation, the more upset I get. In no time flat, my shoulders are up around my ears because all my muscles are tensed from stress. With hunched shoulders, I make my way to the refrigerator, the kitchen pantry, or the cabinet looking for relief. . . . Enough already! The solution is not in there! I've found that when I release the situation, things unfold as they should, and everything works out better than I could have imagined. But I must first let go. So must you. Your heart and your health depend on it.

16

Empty Calories and Other Unnecessary Evils

AS FAR AS DIET BUSTERS GO, depression and resignation are right up there with stress. If you've ever watched an old episode of *Lost in Space*, you will recall the robot flailing his arms and crying, "Danger! Danger!" Yes, depression and resignation are black holes that can be bottomless and lead to nowhere short of foolish choices and hip expansion. Depression and resignation, better known as apathy, don't just affect how you feel, they affect what you do and how you look. The effects of apathy are usually like watching a slow train make its way down an endless track or like watching paint dry. By small degrees our moods and mindsets shift, ever so subtly, that we might not even be aware of it. The sliding scale of sadness to just not caring can be seamless, with no big bumps or alarms—until you go to put your hips into something fitted. Then you realize that you've been wearing layers—literally and psychologically—and elastic for so long that you did not notice the expansion of your waist. Now let me tell you what's really sad—when even the elastic has lost its elasticity and can't stretch to accommodate you anymore. That's when you know "it's on," as they say in the 'hood. Not the fat, but the war is on. It's official that something has to be done. Eh, but here's the dilemma: You know something needs to be done, but apathy makes it hard to care enough to get started. After all, when you've decided you look like a beached whale, what's one more pound at this point?

It happened to me! As I pulled my wardrobe together for a cruise aboard the *Queen Mary 2* luxury liner, I went shopping in my closet for evening gowns only to find out that, unbeknownst to me, my midsection had expanded beyond my wardrobe! Yes, I was the heaviest I had ever been. And for every dress I attempted to zip and then cast to the side when I couldn't get past the middle of my back (don't you wish you could keep the boobs and get rid of the middle?), the truth set in and could no longer be ignored. All those cupcakes had finally caught up with me.

Now, if broccoli had been my drug of choice instead of cupcakes, I wouldn't have had trouble zipping those dresses. But who wants to eat broccoli when you are depressed? Can you imagine? Picture yourself in an emotional slump. Is that the time you say to yourself, "Self, I sure could go for some broccoli, mmm!" Oh, hecky no. You are going to reach for something that has absolutely no substance, no redeeming value, to ease your wounded soul. And I can't blame you! But you cannot continue down this road endlessly, or it is sure to catch up with you—as I found out standing amid a pile of clothing in front of my mirror. Luckily I had a stack of "expandable wear," as I call it. You know what I'm talking about—the elasticized stuff, the crinkled, stretchy stuff, the caftans, all the stuff you ditch first when you feel little and cute. But back to the point.

Cupcakes and empty calories add up to more than a big number. They add up to unwanted pounds that make us feel worse than we were already feeling, and that leads to more depression on a whole other level. Thus the vicious cycle begins, and it can go on indefinitely. So let's deal with depression and apathy for a minute. It's time to unpack this bag and spill the contents. Unless your depression is rooted in physiological issues, such as extreme exhaustion or stress, the root of both depression and apathy comes from a deep place of disappointment—disappointment in whatever. This disappointment can range from the state of your life, to your love life, to your finances, or perhaps just shattered hopes, dreams, and expectations. Disappointment comes from an unfulfilled appointment—a "dissed" appointment, an expectation that was never met or kept. In other words, "hope deferred makes the heart sick."[1] Or, in some cases, it makes you do things to make yourself sick.

Usually when a hope has been deflated, it makes you settle for whatever is within reach. That's why we hear lyrics to songs like "If you can't be with the one you love, love the one you're with." I think this can extend to, "If you can't get what you want out of life, at least you can stuff your face with what you want." Can you say candy bar, little girl? Or fast food? Or anything that is filling but has no nutritional value in it whatsoever?

Empty calories are fillers that do absolutely nothing for you. They just sit there, giving pleasure now but pain and heartache later, kinda' like a bad man. Cute, exciting, but they're not gonna do a thing for you besides being arm candy. Arm candy or candy period—it's time to get rid of both. But you won't unless you know why you chose either in the first place. So let's examine your disappointment and why you've given up hope for a better life, love, or body.

As with any appointment, both people need to know about it. I have found in most cases in which I'm dealing with people who have been disappointed in love, it's because they made an appointment that the other person, their partner, or potential partner, didn't know about and therefore did not keep. In other cases, expectations about life are simply not pragmatic or realistic. They are wild hopes not anchored in anything that promises to deliver what we're looking for. Then we wonder why God has withheld something from us.

In these instances in my own life, I have concluded that perhaps I shouldn't put so much energy into bemoaning what God has withheld from me and instead shift my attitude to be thankful for what He may have saved me from instead. C'mon now, you know what I'm talking about. Just think back to the man you just knew you would die without, and remember your shock the last time you saw him. You knocked yourself in the head and said, "What was I thinking?! Thank you, Jesus, for not letting me end up with him!" But until this revelation comes to light, you might find yourself eating cream puffs, asking yourself why things never worked out with Harry. Or maybe you want to know why things did "work out," and now you're stuck with a man you can't live with and can't kill. Whatever the disappointment, we act it out in ways that are usually not good for us. We find a way to fill the distance in between the wait and the fulfillment of what we crave. And it's usually nothing with substance.

Think of it this way: When you're hungry and on the run, what do you reach for? It's usually nothing that is good. Well, it tastes good, but it does nothing for you. Fast foods, snacks, candy, chips—they load down your system and make you feel full for a little while. Once again, it's kind of like a bad relationship that you know you shouldn't be in. It fills the spot for a minute or a fun evening, but it leaves you wondering what you're doing in the midnight hour when the hunger for a real, good love resurfaces with no commercial interruptions. Empty calories and relationships are the temporary fillers in our lives. Both leave us on E, begging for more.

Usually when I'm in this phase of my life, I wear more oversized things with elastic to hide my sin until I come to myself. I call it being comfortable, but what it really adds up to is lying to myself. You see, if nothing really is fitted, it won't tell me that I'm gaining weight and need to put down my fork and knife. Yes, I can continue my downward spiral into all things bad and fattening as long as my clothing doesn't tell me to stop. Can I get a witness?

Let me give you a heads-up here. Empty calories don't just hide out in bad men and candy. They hide out in stuff that is supposed to be okay, like white rice, white potatoes, refined sugar, processed foods . . . we'll get more specific about these later. Just know for now that these things just take up space and more space and more space, if you get my drift. It's time to seek out the things that have nutritional value. In a relationship, that would be someone who is not only good for you and good to you, but a person who also makes you a better you. In food, it would be foods that not only taste good, but give something back like nutrition, vitamins, and things that make your system healthier and leaner. Foods should give you more than flavor. They should not contribute to your fat ratio. They should add fiber and muscle to your system and inspire your metabolism into burning mode.

When you make a concerted effort to do away with everything in your life that causes you stress and disappointment, you will have to refocus your desires elsewhere. As you learn who is bad for you as well as *what* is bad for you, your tastes should change. At some point you have to make peace with yourself and the mistakes you've made in life, love, and eating and decide that in this moment you can't do anything about what you *did*, but you *can* do something about what you do next. You're not a fool for making a mistake, but you are a fool if you refuse to learn from it and do something differently. So get over it and on with it. That might seem a bit abrupt, but remember, change will never come based on feelings. It will only come when you make a decision to do something about the things you don't like. Repeat after me: "My emotions are to follow my decisions. I am the boss of me!" It's time to clean up your heart and your diet. Get rid of people that drain you and food that is killing you. And for God's sake, get rid of the big clothes and the elastic while you are at it. Stop hiding and come out, come out, wherever you are, no matter what size you are. Here's looking at you, kid. Shake it off and step up. Lift your fist and say, "It's on!"

KEEPING IT REAL

- List the disappointments that affect your outlook on life and yourself.

- Write what expectations were tied to those disappointments. Which expectations were misplaced?

- What fillers became substitutes for what you thought you missed out on?

- Chronicle the changes that occurred in your outlook and habits after you were disappointed.

- Write what things you can take control of right now.

- Write something to be grateful for in the midst of your disappointments. Write an affirmation of your new beginning and how you will move forward.

DIVA REFLECTIONS

One of the things I live by is the exhortation to lay aside every weight and every sin that so easily besets or hinders or weighs and slows us down and run the race with patience and endurance.[2] Every weight is not a sin; it's just not good for you, like an empty calorie. It's hard to be patient with life when you feel out of breath from the weight of the things you've been carrying. I've said it often, but you cannot compartmentalize your character. The choices you make will be reflected across the board. Your emotions, relationships, and eating habits will exhibit similar traits. One undisciplined turn begets another. You will find that, at high-stress times when everything in your world is out of control, your eating will be too. Your home, or perhaps just your bedroom, will be a mess; you will be late to appointments; you'll eat junk food on the run . . . you see where this is all going? Straight south! Life is sure to bring disappointments, upsets, and stresses that are caused by our choices or completely uninvited and unwarranted. The one person you can control in the midst of all the madness is yourself. As you look at life through a big picture window instead of through the keyhole of the immediate circumstance, you will have a clearer view of how to refocus on what is truly important—how you respond in light of your tomorrows. One small decision in the moment, one great step for the rest of your life.

Apples, Pears, and Other Body Types

17

NOW THAT WE'VE DEALT with all the inner workings and things that have been standing between you and the body you want, I would like to focus on getting down to the nitty-gritty of how we are going to be eating from now on. Remember, this plan—although I'll call it the Ultimate Diva Diet—is not a diet! It is a decision you are going to make to die to the way you've eaten in the past. That's right—die to it. I know that for every person who will call Jenny or join some other weight-management program, there are five saying that it's not in their budget 'cause they spent that money on food or shoes or something else to make them feel better. So I am going to share with you a few things I've learned from three "free" eating programs (food combining, eating according to your blood type, and a program that targets your midsection) that I've found to be effective and within my control. The reason I'm going to break down the individual programs I've learned from before I combine them to be the Ultimate Diva Plan for eating and losing is because I want you to be clear on why we are doing what we are doing. Make sense?

The first thing we must acknowledge is that everybody does not have the same body. Every *body* is different. What will work for Mary will not make a dent on Sue. Small wonder you and your girlfriend went on a diet, and she lost twenty pounds to your two. It's enough to make you grab a candy bar and drown your woes of comparison in rich caramel. Hopefully my news will set you free and give you hope. Your body is not everybody's body. God created you uniquely you, which means the way you approach food and even exercise will have to be customized to fit you. Make sense? There are basically three body types: the apple, which means you gain your weight mainly in your upper body, tummy, back, and arms; the pear, which means you gain weight in the hips, thighs, and buttocks; and the banana, which believes in sharing the wealth (or weight) equally throughout the body. Knowing your body type should affect your exercise program; you should place the emphasis on different body parts to maximize the minimum and minimize the maximum. That is an easy enough one to spot. Ah, but then it gets to the not so obvious—the stuff going on beneath the surface.

I discovered the beneath-the-surface issue by accident. During one of my yo-yo periods, I ran into an ex-boyfriend, who sent me off to his nutritionist. When I first met Richard, I was emerging from my latest diet and was a slim goody. As our love grew, so did my waistline. Alas, we went our separate ways but remained friends. After we ran into one another sometime later, he was quite alarmed at my weight gain and health complaints and promptly made an appointment for me to meet with his nutritional guru. After talking with me extensively about all my aches and pains and high cholesterol, the guru introduced me to the concept of eating according to my blood type.

This was revolutionary for me. The nutritionist explained that depending on your blood type and stomach enzymes, you break down and digest food differently, which could affect your health and even the way you gain or lose weight. There are four basic blood types. O is the most popular, followed by A, B, and AB. Once we had figured out that I was an O blood type, he gave me a food chart that listed which foods were highly beneficial. These foods are good and healing for the body. Then there are neutral foods, which means they don't do anything bad—they act like food giving you calories, energy, and fat. Just keep in mind that the beneficial foods actually help you lose weight and the neutral foods don't. Then, there was the list of foods to avoid. These things are actually poison for your system. Well! That list of foods to avoid explained a lot about the way I had been feeling. While I was quietly surprised to find out that I absolutely loved all the food on the beneficial list and neutral list, there were a few things I indulged in on the list of things to avoid. These things, he explained, were probably the source of my struggles with acid reflux, feeling bloated, and being downright gassy at times. Hey, I'm just keeping it real 'cause the truth is the light, my friend.

Since O blood types have been blessed with strong stomach acid and enzymes, we are usually able to metabolize anything, even if it's not good for us, which can lead to problems. I always wondered why I didn't feel so hot after a glass of orange juice. I discovered that was on my avoid list. It is too high in acid. I was supposed to stick to more alkaline fare like pineapple juice or pink grapefruit juice. No lemonade, limeade, apple juice, or orange juice for me! In the past I had noticed that when I went on my three-month strike from eating chicken, I had lost a lot of weight. There was good reason, because chicken is on my neutral list!

I was pleased to find out that blood type O was supposed to eat more red meat. I loved lamb, lean cuts of beef, and fish! Salmon, red snapper, bass—I was in hog heaven but in a good way. I found out why I was lactose intolerant. It didn't jive with my blood type. "If it doesn't fit, don't force it" was a train of thought I had to embrace. Was eating to feel bad really worth it? The answer is no, especially when there were so many things I loved on the list that could make me feel good.

But not just make me feel good. They could actually make me lose weight. Why? Because the body doesn't have to work so hard to break down the food you're shoveling into your stomach. It's important to know that blood type O people are at their healthiest when they stick to a diet that is high in protein and supplemented by fruits and vegetables. In our case, red meat stimulates our metabolism, along with great green vegetables like broccoli and spinach, and some things that may surprise you actually cause weight gain, like brussels sprouts, cabbage, corn, and wheat gluten because they slow down the metabolism.

Blood type A people do better with a mostly vegetarian diet with little or no meat; they don't metabolize meat or dairy well. Things that stimulate weight loss for them are things like vegetables and soy foods, which both metabolize quickly and aid in digestion; pineapple, which helps cleanse the intestines; and vegetable oils, which prevent water retention. For this blood type, meat stores as fat and digests poorly, while dairy and certain beans—such as kidney beans and lima beans—slow down their metabolic rates and interfere with digestion.

All of these things are determined by the thickness of the blood and the levels of acid in your stomach. The authors of the two blood type books (listed at end of this chapter) do a really good job of breaking down which foods are acid versus alkaline in greater detail in their books. Again, I am not a nutritionist. I'm just giving you the basics of what they share, so if you want more details about pH levels, insulin, glucose, high cholesterol, and how the various foods affect your body, I highly recommend you read the books I'm referring to in these chapters. For the sake of where I'm taking you in this book, these are just the abbreviated CliffsNotes. So let's get back to it.

Blood type B people can eat meat and dairy; this is the only blood type that can mix both and thrive. Meat, green vegetables, eggs, and liver all boost their metabolism. The foods that can cause weight gain for them are corn, lentils, peanuts, wheat—these all slow down their digestion and metabolism, causing food to store as fat.

Blood type AB people do well with tofu, seafood, dairy, and green vegetables. All these things stimulate their metabolism and insulin production. The things that cause weight gain are red meat, kidney and lima beans, seeds, corn, and wheat. They do all sorts of bad things such as slowing down the metabolism, messing with insulin levels (which can zap energy), storing fat, digesting poorly . . . get the picture?

It could be safe to say that if we were just sensitive enough to listen to our bodies, we would eat the right things and be fine. But we don't, so that leads to having to spell it out. There are a few simple rules to follow here that go across all blood-type lines. First, try to eat more "live" foods than anything else. That would be things that have not been killed. They are alive—fruits, vegetables, grains. These things have water and fiber that go to work in your system.

When I got home with my list, I called my dad and started relating all the food dos and don'ts to him. This caused him grave concern because the first thing I went after was his white rice. You do not tell an African man he cannot have his rice. I remember, when visiting him shortly after this conversation, telling his cook he was only to be served brown rice and sweet potatoes, and she looked at me as if I were crazy. My dad just couldn't understand. "But why?!" he exclaimed. "The white people get to eat white food," to which I replied, "Well, the black people don't get to eat anything white." This caused him to dissolve into laughter. I then went on to explain to him that all the good stuff has been washed off and removed from white rice. They bleach away all the nutrients. Anything processed or refined just spikes our blood sugars, fakes out our systems, and drops us over the edge, where we crash and are left for hungry again. He wasn't buying it, but I was. I made the switch from white rice to brown rice, from white potatoes to sweet potatoes, from white bread to Ezekiel 4:9 bread, which is packed with live grains.

Helpful stuff to know, right? I call this the first major stepping-stone to permanent weight loss. Of course, you can cross over the line and eat foods you should avoid, but understand the effects and do it in limited measure if you must. You can read more on this subject and find the charts that give you the specific foods for your blood type at the following Web sites:

Blood type O

http://www.drlam.com/blood_type_diet/blood_o_chart.asp

Blood type A

http://www.drlam.com/blood_type_diet/blood_a_chart.asp

Blood type B

http://www.drlam.com/blood_type_diet/blood_b_chart.asp

Blood type AB

http://www.drlam.com/blood_type_diet/blood_ab_chart.asp

Or you can log on to this one address for a brief overview on every type of blood type and downloadable chart for your blood type:

http://pdfdatabase.com/index.php?q=blood+type+food+chart.asp

I highly recommend the following books for a more in-depth understanding for those who need to know every single detail: *Eat Right 4 Your Type* by Peter J. D'Adamo and Catherine Whitney and *Bloodtypes, Bodytypes, and You* by Joseph Christiano. *The Answer Is in Your Bloodtype* by Steven M. Weissberg and Joseph Christiano even gives you menus for if you're active or inactive according to your blood type to help you lose weight.

So this is what I submit to you: For far too long, we have run amuck. It is true. What you don't know *will* hurt you. This is why God says, with all your getting, get an understanding that wisdom is the main thing to strive for.[1] Why? Because we make fatal mistakes when we lack knowledge. No one would deliberately eat a bowl of soup laced with poison. Part of loving yourself is protecting yourself from anything detrimental to your heart, your mind, and yes, your body. As my sister girl Pamela always says, and I've quoted her often, "If people knew better, they would do better." So there you have it. I just dropped some information into your world. Everything that looks good or tastes good might not be good for you. Now you know. Do with the information what you will.

KEEPING IT REAL

- Find out your blood type. (You can get this information from your personal physician or stop by the Red Cross; you could also get your own kit, prick your finger, and voilà, you will know your blood type.)

- Educate yourself on the foods that can help you and the foods that can hurt you.

- Clean out your kitchen cabinets and get rid of the poison.

- Refill your cabinets with things that will feed and heal you.

- Decide to take responsibility for your body like never before.

DIVA REFLECTIONS

As quiet as it's kept, losing weight is not just about the aesthetics. It's about being your personal best healthwise and otherwise. The surface effect is just the natural residual of being in your best state of health. Like water seeking its own level, I think our bodies are trying their best to be what they were designed to be—well-oiled instruments that function at peak performance when we put the right fuel in them. Ah, but we don't let our bodies perform at their best level. We keep settling for low-grade fuel that clogs our engines (bodies) and then wonder why we can't get where we want to go. Let's flip the script on that. Let's be kind to ourselves and listen to our bodies—what they like and don't like (that would be gauged by the body's reaction to what you put in it, not what your tongue tells you). A good body equals a sound mind, sound health, and amazing productivity. Makes sense to me.

Finding the Perfect Combination

NOW THAT YOU KNOW what to eat, let's figure out how to eat it. Keep in mind that I'm going to give you three building blocks I've combined to make how I approach food a complete change of lifestyle versus another painful diet. This is building block two. The theory is simply this: It's not just what you eat but when and how you eat it. Now, before your eyebrows get locked, chill out; I'm going to break this down to the CliffsNotes for you. If you want to read in deep detail what I'm about to unpack, you can pick up a copy of *Fit for Life* by Harvey and Marilyn Diamond. I have tried their advice, and yes, it works. Admittedly, it was hard for me to sustain, and you will understand why once I share it with you. However, I have continued this plan in a modified way that I will share with you later; for now, I will give it to you straight to explain the groundwork of each principle of the Ultimate Diva Diet, so you can understand the rationale behind my directions.

The premise of food combining is based on the natural rhythm of the body and how it works with the food we supply to it. How we eat can assist or hinder the process, which includes appropriation (digesting the food), assimilation (absorbing and using the food), and elimination (getting rid of the food and debris). There are certain times of the day when these three functions are more intense and focused. Appropriation takes place roughly between noon and 8 p.m. Assimilation occurs from approximately 8 p.m. to 4 a.m. And finally, elimination takes place from 4 a.m. to noon. This is the order of food consumption. It is eaten and broken down, and the body divides what it can use from what it can't use and sends the unusable off to be discarded while utilizing what it can use to feed blood, cells, etc. This lifting and separating is going on even when we sleep and should be wrapping up its shift about the time we awake and dash to the washroom. This sounds like a smooth operation, kind of like a factory assembly line. Now picture us throwing a wrench in the middle of this movement. You got it. Everything gets backed up. Stuff starts to putrefy, spoil, harden, cause major problems—like acid reflux, flatulence, gas, bloating, extended colons, and other health problems—especially if you eat late at night. This can throw the whole schedule off if you go to sleep before your body is finished processing your dinner. This is why it is recommended that you eat at least three hours before going to bed. Going to bed on a full stomach is not the way to go. We are all familiar with the effects of that misdemeanor.

Now exactly why is this? It's actually more simple than you would ever think. Here's a quick little science lesson. The body is made up of 90 percent water at birth and decreases to 70 percent water as adults. Small wonder we are encouraged to drink lots of water. Our bodies need to remain hydrated in order to function at their peak. How much water should you drink? The basic standard touted by most is eight glasses a day or roughly sixty-four ounces. This can vary based on hot, humid weather conditions, amount of exertion, etc., as to whether the body might need more or less. There is also the school of thought that you should divide your body weight in half to calculate the number of ounces of water you need to replenish its water content. For example, if you weighed 160 pounds, you would drink eighty ounces of water.

There is also the theory that you can drink too much water and end up with water intoxication, otherwise known as hyperhydration or water poisoning, which can be fatal. This occurs when the normal balance of electrolytes in the body is pushed outside safe limits by overconsumption of water. (But this is an extreme case that happens when you greatly exceed the recommended intake of water.) Consumed in normal quantities, water is good for keeping things moving in your system—for transporting food to all the cells in the body and removing toxic wastes. Basically, water is a natural cleanser and detoxifier, which is hugely important. It is generally believed that those who do not consume enough water are prone to accumulating more body fat than those who do. However, drinking water is not enough.

This is why it is important to not only drink water but to *eat* water in order to replace the water the body expends. Say what? Yes, I said *eat* water. I hear you. "How does one do that?" you ask. By making fruits and vegetables the greater portion of your diet. Fruits and vegetables are high-water-content foods and carry needed enzymes and nutrients into the body. Fruits and vegetables are called unconcentrates. Say that with me now: *unconcentrates*. Why do I want you to become familiar with this word? Because food combining is based on the theory that no human body is designed to digest more than one concentrated food at the same time. Let that sink in. Any food that is not a fruit or a vegetable is a concentrate. That would be potatoes, rice, bread, and pasta— mm-hmm, all that stuff that we are used to mixin' and minglin' together in one meal.

You know I'm a meat-and-potatoes girl from way back! This revelation rocked my world. This was why my system was all clogged up. My poor little body never had the chance to complete a cycle before I was shoveling in another offering it couldn't break down, at least not in the time I gave it to recover. "Now wait a minute," I just heard somebody scream, "potato is a vegetable." That is true, my sister. It is high in water content when it is raw, but once it's cooked, it turns into a concentrate. This continual mixing and matching of concentrated foods makes the body work even harder to break them down. No wonder we get sleepy after we eat those big, heavy meals! We are wearing our poor little systems out. So let me give you a little piece of information that will help you make sense of all this.

Fruit is 80 to 90 percent water, and it contains all the nutrients your body and your brain need to furnish you with energy and cleanse at the same time. Fruit does not stay in the stomach, unless it's a dried fruit or a banana (they take forty-five minutes to an hour to digest). Most fruit passes through the stomach in twenty to thirty minutes, and it's gone! Because of this, it is recommended that you not eat fruit with or after a meal. Oh, I know your hair is on fire now. Visions of all the times you had fruit after dinner in a restaurant or with your cereal are coming back to haunt you. The bottom line? Fruit (we're talking fresh fruit—cooked fruits and pasteurized fruit juices become highly acidic and again, cause problems) should always be eaten on an empty stomach. That way it can go into your system, do what it does, and be on its way. When you eat it with something else, it putrefies, gets stuck, spoils the other food, and causes a lot of bubble, bubble, toil, and trouble in your system. Did I just hear you burp? Keep in mind that some foods are alkaline and some foods are acidic. Depending on your blood type and the acid levels in your stomach, different foods process efficiently or back up and store stuff as fat and create other health problems. Take your pick.

So when can you eat fruit? When your stomach is empty. How will you know when it's empty? Here's the guide: Salads and raw

vegetables take about two hours to make it through your stomach. A meal that has been properly combined without meat (that
would be one concentrate with vegetables, as in penne with tomato
sauce) takes about three hours. A properly combined meal with
meat (such as fish, steamed broccoli, and a salad) would take up to
four hours. And if you really went all out and combined whatever
you wanted to (like you do on Thanksgiving Day), then it could
take a minimum of eight hours to clear out of the stomach.

The Fit for Life program strongly believes that the best time
for fruit and fresh fruit juice is from first thing in the morning
until about noon. This gives the body the opportunity to finish cleansing itself and prepare to digest and break down your
lunch and dinner. This thinking is based on the fact that breakfast
derives from the words *break fast*, as in breaking a fast, which one
should do gently by not overwhelming the system after it has been
resting. After breaking the fast, eating properly combined meals
should add energy to your day without drama and be finished
passing through the stomach before you go to bed. Once the food
passes through the stomach, it is absorbed and broken down in
the intestines, and well, you know the rest. The premise is that the
body doesn't have to work as hard if we work in partnership with
its natural movements.

Obviously the developers of the Fit for Life program lean more
toward a vegetarian diet. They are not big fans of meat or dairy.
They cite that human beings are the only ones that drink milk
after infancy and drink someone else's milk at that. After all, you
won't catch a cow drinking a human's milk or milk from another
animal. This is true, but that's a whole other road to venture down.
I believe that all things in balance are safe. And for those of the
lactose-intolerant persuasion, there are ways to get more calcium.
You can get it in other foods such as greens, fresh orange juice,
beans, soy, tofu, yogurt, white cheeses, oats, almonds . . . the list

goes on. Just know you need calcium; it seems to play its own part in assisting you in weight loss by limiting the amount of new fat your body can make.

Last, but certainly not least, you are going to hate me for this one: Let's talk about coffee for a minute. My masseuse says you should drink two glasses of water for every cup of coffee you consume. The Fit for Life people want you to know that it takes twenty-four hours for a cup of coffee or tea (caffeinated) to get through your kidneys and urinary tract.[1] When you drink coffee with your food, it forces the food to leave your stomach prematurely and slows down the movement of your intestines. Couple undigested food with a slowly moving colon, and what do you get? That's right, constipation! Does decaffeinated coffee make a difference? Considering all the chemicals used to saturate the beans that then go into your system, I say stick with a reduced amount of the real thing, so get a coffee-flavored substitute or switch to herbal tea. This change might be rough for some because, truthfully speaking, caffeine is addictive. It is also a stimulant and can affect your blood-sugar level because it forces the pancreas to secrete insulin. Last but not least, caffeine is acidic. The more acid you have in your blood, the more your body will retain water to try to neutralize it. (By the way, my assistant didn't like this chapter. She said it had way more truth than she was ready to receive. Once again, I'm just delivering the mail. You can do what you will with the contents.)

One more important sidebar—there are a few things that we think of as vegetables that are considered fruits. Avocado, cucumber, bell peppers (green or red), and tomatoes can be eaten with other fruits. So you can combine avocado with papaya, mango, or banana, or cucumber with peaches . . . you got it. These four "fruits" that we think of as vegetables can also be combined with starchy carbs such as bread, pasta, rice, or potatoes. Take note, though, that you should not cook these four fruits. It makes them very acidic. Ever wondered why you burped after those cooked green peppers? had acid reflux after devouring a steaming tomato sauce? Aha! Now you know. Stick to fresh salsa and guacamole.

These are my broad sweeps taken away from what I read about the Fit for Life program and incorporated into my diet plan. I must admit, when following this plan, for the first time, I did not feel stuffed when I ate, I had energy, and I lost weight—so hold on to these thoughts as we move on; they will all come together soon enough.

Again, your body is your body, and my body is my body. This means that, as you absorb all this information, you should be able to be informed enough to understand what your body may have been trying to tell you. Understanding is a beautiful thing. Once you have the basic foundation of where this is going, you will be able to make adjustments according to what your body needs. But the bottom line is that what every body needs is to be fit for life and we're getting there, my sister. We are getting there, one bite at a time.

KEEPING IT REAL

- Write down what you eat every day for a week. Take note of the combinations.

- Write down how you feel after every meal.

- Now try a day where you have fruit in the morning and a nice salad for lunch with some meat. Have another properly combined meal for dinner. Write down how you feel.

- Up your water intake. Cut out soda and lots of juice with added sugar. Try to cut back on the coffee for a week if you can't replace it with herbal or green tea.

- Try this for a week. Journal how your body feels or any changes you notice from eating this way versus the way you ate before.

DIVA REFLECTIONS

It's amazing how much time, effort, and money we spend on our externals and how little dedication we give to what we put into our bodies. We read labels about fabric content, who the designer is, etc., but when it comes to what we eat, how much time do we spend reading labels? Our bodies are the temples that we live in. We need to keep them clean and sound. They're the only ones we get. And just like a badly neglected home deteriorates at a much more rapid rate, so do our bodies. We owe it as a thank-you to God, who created us wonderfully and fearfully, to respect His creation by taking good care of it.[3] We can take our cues from nature. The creatures of nature stay true to who they are. For instance, lions only eat meat. Some animals—depending on their makeup—eat leaves and berries. Animals move a lot and exercise. For the most part, they are lean, mean machines. I realized this with my own sweet little dogs. I had overindulged them with treats when all they needed was their basic food. They, too, had to go on a diet. I found I needed willpower to deny them the things I had taught them to crave. But when I resisted their sad eyes, they lost weight and were happier in the end, minus the extra fat. The same can be true for me and you.

The Right Foundation

PEOPLE TALK ABOUT FINDING their center all the time. You are a spirit that has a soul that lives in a body. Your spirit is your core. When your spirit is anchored and aligned properly, you are able to take all things in perspective and balance your life. The same is true of your body. Your core has to be properly anchored in order for your body to line up and remain strong. Your core is your abdomen. I know some may have thought it was your spine after countless trips to the chiropractor, but a lot of how everything lines up has to do with where you carry your weight. Therefore, you've got to follow your gut to see why some other things in your system are off. So let's talk about building your body from the inside out.

When I got ahold of *The Abs Diet*, a book by David Zinczenko (the editor in chief of *Men's Health* magazine) with Ted Spiker, bells started ringing, and the light came on inside my head. This was the missing piece of understanding for me. Witty, but straight to the point and filled with tons of amazing revelations, this book finally brought all the pieces together for me. David, my new best friend, focused on something that none of the other diets had focused on. While they all had their own ways of making you change your eating habits, cut out certain things, and shave off calories from your diet, none of the plans had shared that our bodies have their own natural fat-burning mechanism—muscle.

David went on to share that building muscle in your body is the key to getting rid of fat and never letting it come back. Muscle speeds up the process of burning fat. We've heard this before, but I didn't know to what extent muscle really affected the body. One pound of muscle requires your body to burn up to fifty extra calories per day in order to keep that muscle.[1] So if you combine exercise with foods that promote muscle growth, you'll turn your fat into muscle, which will then attack the rest of the fat and make you a mean, lean machine.

Now, I heard a collective groan when the word *exercise* came up. I feel your pain, but you knew it had to rear its ugly head at some point, didn't you? The bottom line is that no one will lose weight and keep it off permanently without exercising, but we will talk about this more later. For now, let's get back to the food.

The good part about the muscle revelation is that the "power" foods that build muscle also do some other wonderful things— like make you feel full, give you the nutrients your body needs, and cut your cravings for foods that are not good for you. Whoo-hoo, this is sounding better and better, right?

My new BFF David, with his cute self, went on to share a very simple, basic plan that did not overwhelm me. I had always heard that you should eat three meals a day and two snacks, but Mr. Man said you should eat three meals a day and three snacks evenly spaced out through the day. Hey, I wasn't mad at him for telling me to eat more food, so he would get no argument from me. Snacks were to be eaten two hours before a larger meal. The meals were to be based on twelve food groups and have at least two of the foods from the list (food combining!):

- Almonds and other nuts (not your friends—real, edible nuts, haha!)
- Beans and legumes
- Spinach and other green vegetables
- Dairy (fat-free or low-fat milk, yogurt, cheese—see, I told you everybody wasn't against dairy)
- Instant oatmeal (unsweetened and unflavored)
- Eggs
- Turkey and other lean meats
- Peanut butter
- Olive oil
- Whole-grain breads and cereals
- Extra-protein whey powder
- Raspberries and other berries

All these foods are rich in nutrients and help you get your natural fat-burning mechanism to do its job. This is the stuff that makes you strong and healthy besides looking divalicious. And because David understands human nature, he even gives you one day a week to cheat and eat whatever you want. Constant denial will always lead to bingeing, which defeats the purpose of eating properly.

It was important to focus on eating protein, monounsaturated and polyunsaturated fats, fiber, and calcium. Foods to avoid included refined carbohydrates (stuff that spikes your blood sugar), saturated fats, trans fats, and high-fructose corn syrup.

Why is it called the Abs Diet? Because a good, sound, flat abdomen is at the core of our bodies' health. It is our center. When our abs are strong, they basically set the foundation for our bodies' being in perfect alignment, strengthening our backs and removing stress from our extremities, thus decreasing aches and pains.

When you look like you're carrying a barrel around your middle (say *oo* or *ouch*—whichever works best for you), you are a major setup for trouble. Let's talk about the fact that belly fat is dangerous for the last time. Belly fat releases fatty acids that hinder your ability to break down the hormone insulin (the one that can lead to diabetes if you have too much of it). It also secretes substances that increase your risk of heart attack. It also releases cortisol, that nasty little stress hormone that is associated with heart disease, diabetes, obesity, and high blood pressure. Abdominal fat presses against your liver and your other organs and feeds them poisons while making it hard for them to function under duress.[2] Have I scared you yet? Know that is not my intention; I just want you to be educated about what you are doing to yourself.

But not to worry, I found the Abs Diet program to be a pretty sacrifice-free plan. I still got to eat plenty of the foods I love without craving the wrong stuff because I was too full to miss it. The goal of this plan is to convert the foods you eat into muscle so that the calories you consume go to your muscles to maintain them rather than converting to fat. Isn't that interesting? Muscle actually eats fat! Experts say that a pound of fat adds up to about 3,500 calories. The average woman burns about ten calories per pound of body weight every day just being who she is—without exercise. For every pound of muscle you add to your body, you can burn an additional fifty calories a day (add ten pounds of muscle, and you're burning up to five hundred more calories a day!). That's why we are going to join Diana Ross in singing, "I want muscles!" They don't have to be bulging ones, just cute little ones that keep us looking svelte in that little black dress.

Keep in mind that muscle weighs more than fat, so while you might not see the numbers drop as significantly on the scale, you will see the difference in your body, your midsection, and your clothing. If you're still sitting there saying to yourself, "Well, I'm not that bad," let's do this little exercise together. Check out your body mass index. This will let you know if you're okay, overweight, or obese. Hey, the truth is the light, so let's do this.

To measure BMI log on to http://www.nhlbisupport.com/bmi/bminojs.htm or follow these four steps:

1. Multiply weight in pounds by 703. For example, if you weigh 160, then multiply 160 x 703 = 112,480.
2. Multiply height in inches squared. If you are 5 feet 5 inches (65 inches), then multiply 65 x 65 = 4,225.
3. Divide the answer from step 1 by the answer from step 2. So, 112,480 ÷ 4,225 = 26.6.

In this example, your BMI is 26.6. A BMI of twenty-five to thirty means you are overweight. Thirty or greater is an indicator of obesity. I won't tell you my score if you don't tell me yours.

The other two methods of fine-tuning exactly how you are faring is measuring your waist-to-hip ratio and your body fat percentage. In order to find your waist-to-hip ratio, log on to http://www.healthcalculators.org/calculators/waist_hip.asp or follow these steps:

1. Measure your waist using your belly button as the center.
2. Next measure your hips at their widest point around your butt.
3. Divide your waist by your hips. Example: 35 ÷ 42 = 0.83. You should aim for a waist-to-hip ratio of lower than 0.80, so you would need to lose two inches off your waist.

To configure your body fat percentage, you can usually get help with this at your gym (that is, if you go to one). Between 20 and 31 percent is considered normal. In order to have video-girl abs, your body fat should be about 12 percent. To get a good estimate

of your fat and how much you need to lose, visit http://www
.healthyforms.com/helpful-tools/body-fat-percentage.php or figure it out yourself.

1. Multiply your body mass index by 1.20. Example : 1.20 times
   26.6 = 31.92
2. Then multiply your age by .23. So let's say you are 35 years old.
   That would be: 0.23 x 35= 8.05.
3. Add these two totals together. 31.92 + 8.05 = 39.97.
4. Subtract 5.4 from that number to find your body fat percentage.
   So let's see, here we go—39.97 − 5.4 = 34.57. Based on this,
   you would be about 14 percent over the ideal of 20 percent and
   4 percent over what your goal weight should be.
5. Now to find out how much of your weight is just fat, you would
   multiply your body fat percentage by your current weight. So
   that would be 160 x .35 = 56. That means 56 pounds of your
   weight is just fat.
6. Last step. Multiply your total body fat by the weight goal
   percentage. 56 x .30 = 16, so you need to lose 16 pounds of fat.
   This is not the total of weight you need to lose—just the fat.

Next let's figure out what your weight should be. Log on to
http://www.changingshape.com/resources/references/idealbody
weight.asp, or take the number of inches you are over five feet
and multiply by 5. Add 100 to that. That is your baseline target
weight, but we need to calculate that according to your frame. You
can add 5 to 10 percent more for a large frame; subtract 5 to 10
percent less for a small frame; and stay at the original number for
a medium frame.

David says that, if you are over 133 pounds and you can pinch
two inches of belly fat, you need to lose at least ten pounds from
your current weight; if you can pinch one inch, lose five pounds,

no matter what all your other calculations have told you. Yeah, girl, use your thumb and your index finger and pinch that fat under your belly button.

We have two calculations left. Let's find out your metabolic rate so you can know how many calories your body burns throughout the day on its own. The average for women is one calorie per minute, which totals about 1,440 calories per day. Log on to http://health.discovery.com/tools/calculators/basal/basal.html or multiply your weight by 10 to find out how many calories you need. So 160 x 10 = 1,600 would be your basic calorie needs.

To find out your resting metabolic rate, log on to http://www .shapeup.org/interactive/rmr1.php or take your basic calorie number and multiply by 1.4. (1,600 x 1.4 = 2,240). If you want to lose 1½ pounds a week, you would subtract 750 from that total to see how many calories you can have. Now keep in mind that if you exercise, you get to have more calories. So let's say you do 20 minutes on a treadmill five days a week; multiply 20 by 8 and add to your resting metabolic rate. Plug the numbers in: 160 + (2,240 -750). So the total calories you could have is 1,650. Doesn't that sound better than what you were expecting? If you got lost with all that calculating, log on to http://www.sparkpeople.com to find out not only your basic caloric requirements but also how many grams of carbs, protein, and fat you can have. If you want a more detailed breakdown of exactly how many grams and calories per day, per meal, log on to http://www.shapefit.com/nutrition-calculator.html. (This specific site makes adjustments if you need to do low fat or carbs, etc.) Keep in mind that if you don't do the exercises, you need to consume fewer calories (based on this example you can only have 1,600 calories). I say go for the gold, girl! If you are going to count calories and want to know exactly what your food contains, log on to http://www.nutritiondata.com/. Enter the food you want to know about at the top of the page. It will then let you select specifically what you're eating and then give you all the nutrition facts on it from fat content to glycemic load; you name it, it's all there, my friend, in black and white so you will know exactly what you are putting into your body.

Now that you are armed with all this info (aren't you shocked at how much you didn't know about your body?), hopefully you are ready to get down to serious business. Now I'm going to tell you how I netted out on all of this to incorporate all this great information into the Diva Diet.

I hope by now you've realized that what you don't know can kill you or keep you fat and unhealthy. This is why God says that people err, or should I say make bad mistakes, because of a lack of knowledge.[3] So it's not just your tongue's fault that you are overweight. It's bigger than a lack of discipline or surrender. It simply boils down to everything you don't know about your body, about food and its relationship to how you feel, as well as how your health fares. Now, does that mean that all skinny people are healthy? Lord no, it does not, but we're not worrying about anybody but you right now. The only person you can ever control in life is yourself. This is about you making a decision after everything you've learned to take your body back and transform it into a body that you will love. All right, here we go!

KEEPING IT REAL

- Take a look at yourself in the mirror with no clothes on. Open both of your eyes. Be honest with yourself about what you see and what you need to improve on!

- Take your measurements. Weigh yourself.

- Do the math. Take the time to educate yourself about your body, 'cause knowledge is power.

- Write down the sum of your calculations of your body mass index, body fat, metabolic rate, and how many calories you can work with. Put a sticker with your goal weight in a visible place along with a faith confession of anticipated victory.

- Go through your kitchen cabinets, and do a purge. If it's not a power food, get rid of it. Out with the old, in with the new.

DIVA REFLECTIONS

It's true, what doesn't kill us makes us stronger. The goal here is greater than losing pounds. It's about building stronger bodies so that we are here and available to serve others. I don't know about you, but when I'm feeling sluggish, I become introverted and sedentary, which only heightens my problems, and the vicious cycle of gaining weight and losing out on the best life I could be experiencing begins. As we gaze at the cold, hard facts of what we didn't know and how it set us up for where we are right now, exercising power begins with our making the right choices so that we are able to embrace the power God meant us to have spiritually, physically, mentally, and emotionally. Yes, it all goes together. One thing out of whack has devastating effects on all the others. So raise your hand, and say with me, "Today, I embrace the power I have to take my body back." Now, get ye to the store to stock up on power foods!

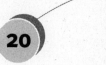

The Ultimate Love Affair

HOPEFULLY BY NOW you've got a made-up mind to do the right thing by yourself and by your body. I have wondered in the past why one of the first great commandments was "Love your neighbor as [you love] yourself."[1] This explains a lot about jealousy, envy, and strife. Apparently, the good Lord knew that we would have difficulty celebrating others, complimenting others, and being genuinely happy for other people's successes. It's hard to love and celebrate others when you can't love or celebrate yourself. When you're overweight, you lack the self-esteem as well as the energy to be active, social, or giving. As you begin to make the right choices and see the results, there will be a transformation emotionally as well as physically. It was so interesting that when my little girl pooch Milan lost two pounds, which is a lot for a dog, she became a whole new dog. She was more outgoing, frisky, and playful. You could tell she not only felt a lot better, but she felt downright cute. It was evident from her new strut and swagger that she knew she was looking hot. It seemed as if every time someone mentioned she had lost weight, she would cock her head to the side and prance a little more! The better she felt, the better she felt about herself and others—a fitting correlation.

The same is true for us. I don't know about you, but when I'm not feeling good about how I look, I tend to agree with the comedienne Mo'Nique, who penned the hilarious book *Skinny Women Are Evil.* But even she has decided for the sake of her family and her health to drop the pounds. The girl is looking good, and now all the overweight sisters that used her as an excuse to stay that way are evil—they feel abandoned. Ah, people—can't live with 'em, can't kill 'em.

At any rate, we are now down to the brass tacks and ready to pull all this information together. I am going to give you my simple formula for what I've termed the Ultimate Diva Diet. I will give you a grocery list, a sample schedule, a sample menu, and a few of my favorite recipes. I am not going to give you a menu for every day because I think that is unrealistic. I have never followed the daily menus in a diet book. You've been eating the way you've been eating for a long time. If I strip you of all that you are used to, you will rebel and binge. Therefore, I am going to trust you to take the good parts of what you love, get rid of the bad parts, and make a few minor adjustments according to my directions in order to come up with your own plan. This plan is about empowering you to make your own choices within the guidelines that I give you so that you can maintain this as a way of life and not return to the mind-set of just following a regimen until you get some weight off. Repeat after me: "I love myself too much to ever go back to where I came from. I am moving forward, never to return to this place." Good girl.

I want you to not eat as if you are fulfilling a duty. I want you to fall in love with the foods you are eating. You've heard the phrase "acquired taste." In some cases, some of you will literally have to acquire a taste for the right kinds of food; you've been eating junk for so long that you and your tongue are convinced that stuff tastes good. I once fell in love with a man who loved sushi. Of course, I learned to love sushi because I loved him. As a matter of fact, my love for sushi lasted long after I had gotten rid of him! It was truly an acquired taste; but once I acquired it, I actually craved it. When I am low on protein, my body will scream out for sushi. I have laughed and called it my new drug of choice. Now it's one of my favorite foods.

I have to confess to you that as I started doing all my research for this book, the more I read, the more I got downright grossed out! The more I discovered what certain things were doing to my body, I developed a deep distaste for them. On the flip side, I began to rediscover some things I hadn't eaten in a long time and to revel in the flavor of them. All of a sudden broccoli was absolutely delicious! Natural, unsweetened peanut butter, cottage cheese, avocado, and tomato slices with just a splash of olive oil and a dash of sea salt— mmmmm! I was amazed at the robust flavors of basic foods unadulterated by a bunch of processing. The thing I love about eating in places like France and Italy is their insistence on fresh foods and clean and simple flavors. When something is creamy, it is creamy on purpose—not because they're trying to cover up the fact that the flavor has been cooked out of something. As much as the French love their food and spend copious hours eating and "conversating," they remain svelte for the most part because of their approach to food: fresh, unadulterated, small portions. All things in moderation (sounds biblical to me), eaten slowly—thus all the endless conversation. In places like France and Italy, it is not just about eating. The dining experience is communion. Perhaps this is why they eat so little and feel full. They are so busy talking in between bites that the stomach actually has the time it needs to register that it doesn't need any more food. But in America, we seem to shovel food down so fast, the body doesn't have time to go, *Whoa, I've had enough!* The body is just scrambling to sock it away and make room for the rest of what is coming!

When you take the time to have a love affair with your meal—as in the sense of being present and aware of the flavors and truly enjoying them—your satisfaction level will peak a lot faster than if you're just throwing your food back. Your tongue wants to have the experience of tasting, and the body wants the luxury of digesting at its natural pace instead of being hurried along. So sit, taste, savor, enjoy, and revel in the respite that eating a good meal provides. Do this even with snacks—don't just down those nuts; chew them, feel the texture, the rich flavor. When you take your time, the stomach sends signals of being full to the brain. That's when you have an experience of complete satisfaction, thus fulfilling your hunger for those dreaded empty calories. Soon, you will be able to treat them like bad men that you no longer need or, more important, want.

So . . . on to the plan. Hopefully by now, you've cleaned out your kitchen cabinets. I am going to give you a list of things you need to get to replace all those bad lovers in your life that promised you good feelings and left you worse for the wear. These are a few staples that have become a part of my life forever because they love me as much as I love them, or perhaps more. I know they will love you, too.

We will take these in order of David's list of power foods (you remember him . . . the Abs Diet guy). Keep in mind, however, that you should also be armed with your blood-type chart so that you select the right foods according to your blood type, which I will refer to as your BT list from now on.

Nuts and seeds—raw, unsalted—A yummy snack and great on salads, they are high in protein, calcium, and natural oils. But don't go overboard! Eat small quantities. (Since people need boundaries, stick to an ounce a sitting—that does not mean ten sittings a day!) Pumpkin, sunflower, sesame, and poppy seeds are great for munching or on top of salads. Just don't mix with another concentrate if you do them on salads. Two tablespoons of flaxseed every day on top of yogurt, or in your protein shake, is a great way to add some fiber to your diet. If you struggle with high cholesterol, it is believed to help lower it.

Beans and legumes—You can get them dried, fresh, or frozen. Fresh is first preference. Please, please, please grow to love edamame if you don't already. It is so good for you. These little soybeans are a natural source of estrogen and are packed with great nutrition, protein, and fiber; they also protect against heart disease. Plus, they are tasty!

Vegetables—Again, fresh is first preference. Your green vegetables are especially potent—broccoli, asparagus, spinach (there was a reason Popeye had to have his spinach . . . you need yours, too). Pay attention to vegetables with intense color. Beets, carrots, bell peppers—they're not just pretty, but they are intensely good for you!

Dairy (fat-free or low-fat milk, yogurt, cheese)—If you are lactose intolerant, lactose-free milk, yogurt, and the white cheeses are going to be your best bet (yellow cheeses are dyed). There are also great milk alternatives: soy, rice, and almond milk—all are delicious without the lactose drama and have great health benefits. Make sure you supplement with calcium supplements if you don't eat enough in this section. Try to stick to plain cow's or goat's milk yogurt.

Oatmeal or the right kind of cereal for your blood type that has high roughage and fiber—Oatmeal is considered a "good" carb because it is a complex carbohydrate. It reduces cholesterol and maintains your blood-sugar levels. If you can't have oatmeal, try another high-fiber cereal like Kashi, All-Bran, or Fiber One. Stay away from cereal with sugar or high-fructose corn syrup.

Eggs—Try the organic ones, with the brown shell; eggs are high in protein and low in calories. If you have high cholesterol, consider eating only the egg whites and leaving the yolks alone.

Lean meats—Yes, lady, you have a lot of choices here besides chicken and turkey. Let's see, there are lean cuts of steak, lean ground beef, lean pork loins, lamb for the type O people, and I recommend Canadian bacon instead of conventional bacon because it has a lot less fat. Of course, fish is great for you; it is nice and lean with good oils that are helpful to you. Load up on the fish, and keep the other meats in balance.

Peanut butter—There is a nut butter for every blood type, so if peanut doesn't agree with you, there are almond, cashew, sesame, and sunflower. These are wonderful for snacks with raw vegetables. Two teaspoons for dipping celery, carrots, jicama . . . yum! Again, don't go crazy here and cross the line to fattening. Try peanut butter in your protein shake; it tastes like ice cream!

Olive oil—The debate goes on about if you should cook with olive oil. If you do, make sure it is cold pressed and minimally processed and refined. (Extra virgin is cold pressed.) Olive oil is more beneficial healthwise served cold on salads, as a bread dip instead of butter, etc. Other oils to consider are almond, avocado, and safflower. Sesame and coconut are usually suggested because they react well to heat and are less perishable after heating. Coconut should be used sparingly, but it is delicious!

Whole grains, gluten-free breads, and cereals—I highly recommend Ezekiel 4:19 bread and Essene bread. Considered "live grains," they can be found in the refrigerator at the grocery store. They are robust, flavorful, and filling. Wasa Crispbread, Finn Crisps, rice cakes, and kasha are all good stuff. (Check your BT chart to see what's best for you.) Across the board, stick to brown and whole-grain breads. These are again "good" carbs that prevent you from storing fat. Let's face it: You need carbs. They're like men; there are still some good ones out there . . . so make sure you choose the right ones.

Stick to brown or wild rice. For flours and meals—stick to cornmeal, rye flour, whole-wheat flour. Remember, we are avoiding refined things that have been stripped of their nutrients and replacing them with things more natural and higher in fiber.

Extra protein—Get extra-protein whey powder—this is one of your main power foods. Protein whey isolate boosts your immune system. Have a protein shake midmorning or a half hour after you've had your fruit. Have one at night, too. Protein shakes keep you from getting hungry and ensure you receive the highest quality protein for your body. A protein shake at night slows your insulin production and allows you to access body fat for energy while you sleep. It's called burning fat while you sleep. I'm all up for that . . . or is that down for that? Sweet dreams!

Berries—Who knew those pretty little things had so much power? Considering they're packed with antioxidants, fiber, and vitamin C, you just got to love 'em! Raspberries, blueberries, strawberries—again they taste just *mahvelous* in your protein shake; or sprinkle a smidgen of raw brown sugar over them (just a smidge!), leave in the refrigerator overnight, and eat the next day . . . or put in the blender to make a nice jam to spread on your Ezekiel 4:9 bread . . . it's so good that you'll want to slap a stranger! Of course, these berries don't need any help, so you can always eat them as is.

Fruit—In general, all fruits are good for you. Eat a lot of them, and they will keep your craving for sweets at bay. Just remember to eat them clear of anything else unless it is a vegetable fruit. There is high praise from most diet experts for grapefruit; it is alkaline and works well with all blood types. Fruits high in water content are more filling and lower in calories, so try watermelon, honeydew, cantaloupe, apples, pears, you get the picture. You can freeze them as balls or chunks for a refreshing, natural popsicle or throw them in the blender for a delicious fruit frosty. Eat dried fruits such as figs, raisins, and mango in small quantities, and make sure they are sun dried.

A few more things:

Sweet potatoes instead of white potatoes—Higher in fiber and better for you.

Pastas—Vegetable pastas, whole wheat, sesame (the natural ones with more grains) are top choice. Remember, we want to eat foods that keep our bodies working!

Snacks—Stick to things that are not loaded down with salt or sugar. Want some chips or something crunchy? Try kettle chips (unsalted) or air-popped popcorn minus the butter and salt. Sprinkle your snacks with an herb substitute for flavor.

Salt substitutes—Bragg Liquid Aminos, sea salt, soy sauce, and Spike are all free of MSG. My favorite is Benson's Gourmet Seasoning. It is an all-natural herb combination that tastes like salt. Log on to www.BensonsGourmetSeasonings.com for more info.

Sugar substitutes—Maple syrup, maple sugar, date sugar, raw cane sugar, and raw honey are some good ideas. I used to really like agave (a yummy sugar substitute made from the agave plant, a form of cactus), but there have been some recent studies suggesting it is highly processed—so be careful and read every label before you buy a product. Basically, stick to the real thing. The body knows what to do with the real thing, but it has no idea how to break down the fake stuff. So if you are going to do sugar, then do it in its natural form. Remember, whatever the body can't break down gets stored as fat or becomes a health problem eventually. Plus all the sugar pretenders mess with you psychologically to make you believe you can eat more because you're not having sugar—liar, liar, pants on fire! And one note about honey: When it's heated over 130 degrees, it becomes acid and useless to the body. Stevia is a natural sugar substitute if you are insistent on avoiding real sugar.

Stock up on lemons—They're good in a glass of room-temperature water first thing in the morning, and they add zest to veggies.

Salad dressings—Look for the ones that don't have sugar, vinegar, or chemicals. I'll give you a recipe to make your own later. Also look for mayo that is low fat with no sugar.

Teas—This drink is much better for you than coffee. Stock up on green tea (it's supposed to be a wonderful aid to weight loss), white teas, and herb teas. Peppermint and ginger are wonderful and aid in digestion when they're natural. You can boil down mint leaves or a branch of ginger yourself and add the concentrate to water for a lift anytime.

Hopefully I've given you enough information for you to now create your own list based on your blood type and what appeals to your taste buds. This should be a liberating exercise now that you see you have more options than you thought. Yeah, girl, the road is narrow, but there is a lot of liberty on that road. Making the right choice versus the wrong one frees you to enjoy the choices you make and to live a better quality of life. As we move on, I will tell you how we are going to combine all the things you've learned into a simple plan you can follow without a lot of angst. First, I want you to embrace the fact that you love yourself enough to change your regime and be good to yourself. When you love your body, it will love you back. Remember, it's the only body you get. There will be no trade-ins, and overhauls could be painful and ineffective. So let's wise up and eat right!

KEEPING IT REAL

- As you go over your blood-type chart, make a note of all the things you already naturally enjoyed eating, and give your body credit for having the sense to know what's good for it.

- Make a new basic grocery list for yourself. Highlight your favorites!

- Make a list of your weaknesses that are not good for you so that you get a clear resolve to stay away from these things. Write *AVOID* in big red letters over your list.

- Get creative with old staples, and find new, exciting recipes to add zest to meals.

- Develop a new mind-set about how you are going to approach food. Write down a positive confession about your new attitude and new love. No more empty calories for you. A healthy body makes a healthy mind and mind-set.

DIVA REFLECTIONS

I believe the ultimate love affair is that you love your Creator enough to take care of the gift He gave you—that would be your body. It is on loan to you. He entrusted you with it. Consider how you would feel if you left a treasured gift in someone's hands. When you returned to claim it, you found it bloated, scarred, and broken. How disappointed would you be? When we receive something from someone that we love, we treasure it because we are aware that it was given in love. Trust me on this one. The One who formed you in your mother's womb considered you an amazing work of art.[2] As a tribute to the artist, we should care for His amazing creation (that would be our bodies)—with love. So take a moment to ask God to forgive you for abusing your body and not appreciating the gift He gave you. He's always willing to forgive. And then, forgive yourself. Promise to be kinder to you and to relax; it's hard to do anything under duress and stress. A little love can go a long and lovely way.

All Things Are Lawful

IT IS ONLY AFTER OUR MINDS have been renewed that we can hope to see our lives or our bodies being transformed. This is not the time to be double minded. No more cramming all the stuff that we know is not good for us into one sitting to wish it good-bye, uh-uh. Our change begins today, not tomorrow, and as President Obama has been quoted to say, "We are the change we've been looking for." It's true, 'cause after we have called Jenny and everybody else, we are going to have to live with ourselves. We can rise up to eat and play and take no thought of the consequences, or we can finally grab the bull by the horns and say enough is enough! All things are lawful, but they are truly not beneficial. It is important to do, eat, and enjoy all things in moderation. What does that mean? You can eat everything you have always eaten—just not as much or just not every week or every day, depending on what it is. Know your weaknesses, be honest with yourself, and set the right boundaries.

An old preacher said many years ago, "Since I got saved, I smoke as many cigarettes as I want, carouse with as many women as I want, and get drunk as much as I want. The problem is that I just don't want them anymore." In other words, he was now able to say no to things that once held him captive. The truth will set you free, and that's why I spent most of this book dwelling on it.[1] Hopefully by now, you feel the same way I do. All right already! I'm never going to overindulge in any of that junk again, so let's get it on!

So what is my Ultimate Diva Diet? It is a combination of the principles from the last three diets I spent time elaborating on. I highly recommend that you check out the books from each one to get an in-depth understanding of the things I shared. As I said, I am not a doctor or a nutritionist; I am a woman just like you in search of what works, and this is what works for me. I am not going to make grandiose claims that you will lose twelve pounds in two weeks or twenty pounds in a month. This is not a sprint. Your new eating habits need to be a steadily paced marathon that goes the distance. Slow and steady wins the race, à la the turtle and the hare. We've been to that country (you know, Lose It Quick, Fast, and in a Hurry), taken the pictures, and come back home with all the pounds we lost and more. We're not going back there again. This is the skinny on losing it and keeping it off. It took you some time to pile on all those extra pounds, and it's going to take some time to take them off.

Someone was admiring the fabulous Heidi Klum (you know, my *Project Runway* girl I mentioned in chapter 4); the admirer was gasping in awe over how quickly Heidi was in shape to model for Victoria's Secret just four weeks after having a baby. The woman was wondering how she could get her body back after having her baby, like Heidi did. Heidi asked her what she looked like before she got pregnant. (Got the point?! You've got to be realistic about your goals.)

We are going to set realistic goals so you don't get discouraged. Keep in mind that the more weight you have to lose, the faster it will fall off initially, and then you will plateau. As your body catches on to what you are doing, it will make adjustments, so it is important for you not to get in a rut or routine with what you eat or even how you exercise. Mix it up, and have fun. Don't be predictable. Remember, if you keep it interesting, you will continue to have fun and not feel denied. If you need an extra jolt during this time to get past your plateau, *The 4 Day Diet* by Dr. Ian Smith gives some great guidelines and food combinations to help you break through. It is all in keeping with what I've shared. (I have a crush on him, too. Call me fickle.)

When your weight plateaus severely or you find yourself perpetually stuck at the same place, you may need a more dramatic form of help to get past where you are. There are several options you can try if a cleanse or a jump-start food plan does not work for you. Your problem could be hormonal, or your body could literally be resisting losing weight based on any number of issues. You can discuss this with a doctor who specializes in hormones or natural weight-loss treatments. Two ways I've known people to deal with stagnant weight loss are acupuncture or HCG (Human Chorionic Gonadotropin), an aid to jump-start your system. I had an assistant who could not lose weight, no matter what she did. The poor girl was practically starving herself to no avail. She went the acupuncture route to trigger her metabolism and began to lose weight. Another assistant I had also could not lose weight and used HCG. HCG tricks the body into thinking it is pregnant, mobilizes stored fat, and suppresses the appetite in order to get the body to start dropping the weight it's been holding on to. It comes in the form of self-administered shots or liquid. She had dramatic results. You can log on to hcgdietinfo.com and check out Dr. Simeon's Weight Loss Protocol as well as Kevin Trudeau's book *The Weight Loss Cure* if you're stuck and want to learn more about this. Again, I think this is if all else fails, and it should not be done without thorough consultation with your doctor. Otherwise be patient with yourself and celebrate consistent and steady weight loss.

The key is all things in moderation. The average healthy weight loss is about 2 to 2½ pounds a week. So underpromise and over-deliver. Let's set the goal at one pound a week—a pound that we are going to get off and keep off. That way you won't feel bad if you only lose a pound, and you will be really excited if you lose more. No pressure means more consistent success.

The first thing I want you to do is what I call "Stripping Your Palate." That's right, we've got to cleanse your palate of its over-the-top craving for sweet things and recalibrate it to want "good" sugars. Those would be the ones found naturally in fruits and fruit vegetables. Therefore, we will begin with a fast. There are several types of fasts that you can do. If you're really brave, you can try the twenty-one-day regimen I mentioned earlier, or you can do liquids only for three days, add fruit only for two days, ease in vegetables for four days, ease back in grains for three days, and finally add meat. Remember, you will only eat fruit on an empty stomach. Have as many fruits and vegetables as you want during this time. And drink plenty of water. If you can't do the liquid-only days, then do three days of fruit only and then add your vegetables, etc. This sets the stage for getting rid of the toxins and garbage in your system. If you want to, pick up a gentle colon-cleanse system from your local health food store to move things along; but if you're eating all those fruits and vegetables, you should have no problem unless you are seriously impacted and irregular from past bad habits. There is a very gentle laxative tea called Smooth Move that I recommend you drink at night for three nights. It is exactly that, but it does the job.

Now that we've recalibrated our taste buds, we can move forward. Across the board, the basics of a good balanced diet include a bit of everything in different measures. Remember, you need to eat three meals and two to three snacks every day. This should include two servings of dairy, two to three servings of 2 to 3½ ounces max of protein, at least two fruits, and lots of vegetables. The things that are going to keep you feeling full are fiber and protein. Your protein servings should be about 2 to 3½ ounces, which is about the size of your cupped palm. Space out your meals according to what you have combined if you want to eat fruit during the day. It is important for you to eat often, but keep your portions small. If you're eating properly, you will eat smaller portions anyway because you will be full faster.

So let's take a look at a few sample menus. Remember, we are staying mindful of how we combine our food. I will give you a menu following the Fit for Life (FFL) formula[2] and then a more generic menu for those of you who believe you have to have more than fruit for breakfast. Either way, you will lose weight. I highly recommend the FFL approach for those who struggle with indigestion and staying regular.

I recommend starting every day with a glass of room-temperature water with some fresh lemon. It is both refreshing and cleansing. Some recommend a little apple cider vinegar, but vinegar is not good for all blood types.

BREAKFAST
- Grapefruit or fruit salad or a fruit smoothie with protein
- Nice herbal tea

SNACK
- Fruit or fruit juice—If you feel you need something with a little substance, try freezing fruit slices and adding them to your drink or blending them into a frosty.

LUNCH
- Salad with some sort of protein (beans, eggs, chicken, fish . . .) or

- Vegetable sandwich
- Vegetable soup

SNACK
- Celery sticks with nut butter or
- One ounce of nuts

DINNER
- Steamed fish
- Sautéed vegetables
- Salad (don't overdo the dressing!)
- Peppermint tea

SNACK
- Fruit with fruit sorbet or protein shake

Of course, it's a given that you need to drink water throughout the day. You may also have as much herbal tea as you like. If you drink more than one cup, learn to enjoy it without sugar or other sweeteners. Besides being mindful of what you eat and how you combine it, be diligent about cutting back sugar to the bare minimum, along with salt. Remember, your last meal should be eaten three hours before you go to sleep.

The next menu is for those of you who balk at not being able to have a more traditional breakfast. In this case I suggest that you still have a piece of fruit, preferably a pink grapefruit or melon, a half hour before you have your breakfast.

BREAKFAST
- Grapefruit (a half hour before everything else . . . so enjoy and then prepare your breakfast)
- Two eggs, sliced tomatoes

SNACK
- Slice of Ezekiel 4:9 bread with hummus or a protein shake

LUNCH
- Mixed greens and tuna salad

SNACK
- One ounce of nuts, half cup of fat-free yogurt (add a touch of honey—delicious)

DINNER
- Vegetable soup, grilled lean meat, salad, or steamed veggies
- Snack
- Fruit, frozen fruit sorbet, or a protein shake

Notice that each meal incorporates protein to keep your system burning. If you keep your meals simple, you can still have all the flavors you crave, just not at the same time. Remember, you can have as many vegetables as you want and a minimum of two fruits a day. The goal is to have at least five servings of fruits and vegetables a day.

There is a plethora of snacks you can have:

- Air-popped popcorn—A 1/4 cup, unpopped, is one hundred calories.
- String cheese—not the whole pack, one at a time please
- Low-sodium V8 juice
- Whole-wheat crackers (just a couple)
- Energy bars—Check the contents; try to stay away from the ones loaded with sugar.
- Low-fat yogurt
- Fat-free pudding
- Unsweetened applesauce—Add a drop of agave if you must or blend with a sweeter fruit.

Choices abound. As you become familiar with portion sizes and pace yourself, you will feel satisfied but not stuffed, within safe boundaries but not denied. Stick to the rule of one for things with more fat, like slices of cheese, etc. That means one fat-free brownie—the absence of fat does not give you permission to have two. So you'd have one tablespoon of spread, one ounce of pasta, one tablespoon of mayo or nut butter or butter. Keep cereals and grains at ¾ to 1 cup, things high in sugar like corn to ½ cup. These are rough calculations per one hundred calories. You can log on to http://www.my-calorie-counter.com if you want to count calories more accurately. If you have an iPhone, you can download several apps to record what you're eating and how it's adding up. This is bondage to me, so I prefer a more organic experience where I feel free to choose the right portions without obsessing over numbers. I never was good at math.

As a matter of fact, to guarantee smaller portions (without doing all the calculations), I suggest using a salad plate instead of a dinner plate to put your meals on. When out at restaurants, order an appetizer portion as opposed to an entrée. Do this until your system becomes used to smaller portions and automatically knows when to stop. Remember my skinny-people observance? They seldom order more than they can eat, or they leave half of their food on their plates. If you can control yourself and you really want the entrée portion, eat only half. Take the other half home, and have it for lunch another day. That way you won't feel as if you are missing anything.

The key to being successful with this information is making your own menu for the week, being mindful of your combinations and food choices. (It's good to keep a food diary, anyway, because it keeps you on track, trust me.) When the facts are there in black and white on the page looking up at you, there is no argument. I have a friend I was holding accountable on her weight-loss journey. She had to e-mail me what she ate every day. When she didn't report her meals to me, she gained weight. 'Nuff said. It's called planning your work and working your plan, by holding yourself accountable.

Pick an evening to prepare your food for the week. I love those Glad containers. I portion out my meals in those and stock up my lunch and my snacks for each day (that's right, I have my apples cut up or whatever I'm having put together for easy access). On my way to the office, I grab my food for the day and am able to stay on track because I'm not left wandering around eating the wrong things when I don't have the right ones within ready reach. Try to keep your caloric intake between 1,400 and 1,600 calories a day initially. As you build more muscle and lose more weight, you will be able to increase it and still lose weight. If you can, do an all-fruit-and-salad day once a week. This gives your body a fasting day for cleansing and rejuvenation. It also keeps you in a lean mind-set. And don't forget—water, water, and more water.

Last but not least, take a good multivitamin. When your body is starving for nutrients, it sends you in search of food. A multivitamin will balance your hunger and help you not to overeat.

Well, that's basically it! It's not as complicated as you think. It boils down to very simple things: what you eat, how you eat, and how much you eat (portion sizes). This is not about starvation. It's about eating what you need as opposed to everything you want. Your wants can fall within your needs with boundaries that ensure your health and the body you want. Remember, you are not a prisoner of your body. You are the warden. You are the boss of you. Take your power back, and handle your business! No more volunteering to be a victim of the foods you are eating. You are going to make choices that serve you—serve your satisfaction and good health. And that, my friend, is a beautiful thing.

KEEPING IT REAL

• Dust off that food journal if you haven't been using it, and get diligent about chronicling your journey. Make it fun. Write funny stories about your experiences and thoughts.

- Write the things that will be most important for you to remember so that you internalize your game plan.

- Write your menu for the week.

- Prepare and portion out your rations.

- Take your time eating, and enjoy your food!

- If you're the type of person that forgets to eat, set the alarm on your phone to remind you to eat something every three hours.

- Don't weigh yourself more than once a week.

- Concentrate on feeling good, and let your body do the rest.

- Give yourself permission to have whatever you want one day a week, but keep it under control. Remember, this is not about denial; it's about you mastering your appetite until it lines up with what you know is best for it.

DIVA REFLECTIONS

We have more power than we know. We have the power to make a difference in how we feel and look. It all boils down to one small word—*decision*. Decide what you want to look and feel like, and decide what you are going to do about it. We have been given the power to choose life or death, blessings or curses every day. I urge you to choose life. Choose to live life wisely. Choose to live in a way that begets life—not only to yourself, but to others. Many of you reading this are mothers. You get to set the example for your children so that they don't experience the same struggle now or later in life. Many have succumbed to diseases and conditions that are believed to be hereditary. In lots of cases, changing the way we eat can save us from a lot of sorrow, pain, and medical bills. The responsibility is ours. Let's take it and run with it, all the way to a more beautiful and healthy you.

22

Move It, Sister!

UNDERSTAND AND KNOW before we even begin this discussion that I hate, hate, hate exercise. Did I say hate? Yes, I did! Unfortunately, no diet on earth works without it, especially if you're over thirty, so get over the idea that, while you cut back on eating, God is going to come down and wave a magic wand over you while you sleep and you will hop up miraculously thin. It won't happen, girlfriend, so you are going to have to get yourself moving. Get your happy self on somebody's treadmill, bike, whatever your preference—you've got to shake it up. Put on some dance music and get in the groove, but you have got to get that heart to pumpin', get to jumpin', and shake that fat off!

I've said it a million times: Attitude is everything. I have two friends, Miss Dee Dee and Tracy Lynne. These two sisters will put you to shame. They are obsessed with working out. Both of them have the cutest little bodies you ever want to see. I just grit my teeth and say "Praise the Lord" every time I see them. The biggest crisis for them is not being able to get a workout in—you would think the world had come to an end because they didn't get to exercise on a given day. Can you believe it? You name it, they do it. Kickboxing, yoga, spin class (that's something they do with bikes I won't be attempting anytime soon). They thrive on it. They insist it gives them more energy. And that is the truth. I have learned that, if you always feel tired, you are not moving enough. Energy begets more energy, and that energy burns fat.

So let's hash it out when it comes to exercise. I'm going to challenge you because I've managed to finally get into the exercise groove too. I dug my treadmill out of my sister's basement and put it at the foot of my bed so I would have to trip over it to get past it. All it took was for one of my male friends to tell me my treadmill was going to end up as a clothes rack to make me determined to prove him wrong. So now, while I watch my favorite programs that I've TiVoed (*Project Runway*, *Top Chef*, *So You Think You Can Dance*, and *Sherri*), I just walk and watch. After that, I use my bands and do some resistance exercises, and finally I graduate to the floor for a set of abdominal reps. I've got to tell you, the first thing I noticed after I got in an exercise routine was that my sleep became more regulated. I slept better and woke with a burst of energy instead of dragging myself out of bed ready to throw a shoe at somebody. I have made a covenant with myself that I must do something for at least twenty minutes every day. I give myself one day a week off—that would be Sunday—and then on Monday, I hit it again. If I get thrown off and something comes up during the week when I don't exercise, I consider that my day off and work out on Sunday. I make sure I move my body more than usual at least six days a week.

Now that I'm getting up earlier, I've moved at least getting on the treadmill to the morning, which is actually better. When you work out on an empty stomach, it gets your metabolism going, so when you do eat, the calories get burned up right away because your body needs them for energy. Some trainers believe that, if you eat right after working out, that meal gets burned up right away.

One of my favorite things to do is a DVD set I discovered a few years back. My sister and her husband got on a roll with it, and the results were dramatic—so dramatic in fact that my sister won their before-and-after contest for results. They flew her to Hawaii to be a part of their next infomercial! Yeah, girl, my sister is on TV. The girl went from a size ten to a size four! She was a lean, mean machine, and her husband was looking all buff. So I got hold of the DVD and started doing the routine, and I, too, could see the difference after about four weeks. The name of the DVD set was Power 90, part of the Beachbody series. Log on here for more info and to get your own copy: http://www.beachbody.com/product/fitness_programs/power90.do. They also have a program called Slim in 6 that is effective, but Power 90 is my favorite. It incorporates different types of exercises in a thirty-five-minute program. Everything from cardio to boxing, kickboxing, yoga, and ab work. It's fun because everything is done in sets of five minutes, so you don't get bored or tired of the exercises. Because the exercises localize specific areas of the body, it fires up all the muscles and makes them lean and strong without looking bulky. You feel strong, and your clothing begins to hang differently in a matter of weeks. If exercise is not your thing, try Zumba. It incorporates Latin and Caribbean dancing to whittle away the inches, and it is a blast. The music is outrageous, and you almost feel like you're having too much fun to be doing anything significantly good for your body, but you are. The dances target abs, glutes, thighs, and arm muscles. Who said the road to looking good could be this much fun?! And last but certainly not least, add Wii Sports to the mix for some virtual exercise fun that works up a sweat that once again doesn't feel like the dirge of normal exercise.

It doesn't take long to shape up if you are doing the right thing. Halle Berry told Oprah when she was training for her part in *Catwoman* that she worked out thirty-five minutes a day. I have had results by working out thirty-five minutes consistently. I warm up on my treadmill for ten minutes, then do my strength and resistance exercises for about twenty to twenty-five minutes, or I do my Power 90 DVD for thirty-five minutes. On days when I am not doing those floor exercises or the DVD, I walk on the treadmill for twenty to sixty minutes (never less than twenty, more if I get caught up in a show I'm watching) as time allows. Consistency is the key. When your body figures out that you have decided to be active, it will cooperate with you and line up. So commit to a time frame that won't make you keep putting it off.

I think one of the things that scares people away from exercising is not only the hatred of sweating but the actual time it takes away from the tyranny of the urgent in your already busy life. But let me tell you this: You cannot afford not to do four things in life—exercise, pray, read the Bible, and tithe to God (giving 10 percent of your income to the Lord) and to yourself—that means saving money or putting a portion of your income aside for retirement, emergencies, goals, etc. These are solid investments that ensure your well-being physically, mentally, emotionally, and financially. They feel inconvenient but reap huge dividends. Again this goes back to loving yourself and your body and giving it what it needs. Besides burning fat, you need to exercise to keep your muscles, your core, and your extremities strong. I have a lot of trouble with my knees, but when I exercise and build up the surrounding muscles, I have less joint pain. So exercise for the sheer selfishness of feeling better.

How you go about it is up to you. You can go to a gym if you like community exercising. As you know, you can go anywhere from the YMCA, which has very reasonable rates for using their workout facilities, to the "she-she, pooh-pooh, la-la" places where all the beautiful people go. I like the comfort of my own home, and the results can be just as achievable. All you need is a mat, a set of exercise bands, and an exercise ball, and you're good to go. There is a plethora of DVDs to help you work out too. You can Walk Away the Pounds, get intense with Billy Blanks, Turbo Jam, you name it. Just make sure that you are not *just* doing cardio. Cardio will burn fat, but it won't build muscle, and muscle is what is going to solidify your weight loss. Try to switch up your routine so that your body doesn't get used to one set of anything. So every other day, consider doing cardio (bicycling, walking, etc.). The other days you should focus on weight lifting or resistance training that works out a specific area of your body.

The first day my trainer, Victor (with his gorgeous self! when I'm not hiding from him he's good to look at . . .), has me do an upper-body day that focuses on my chest, shoulders, biceps, and abs. The second day working out, he focuses on my lower body—calves, hamstrings, inner and outer thighs, and quads. On the third workout day, he has me work out my upper back, triceps, abs, and lower back, with intervals of cardio in between for five to ten minutes. We always start with a warm-up on the treadmill for about ten minutes, then begin and end with stretching. Don't want to shock your muscles or hurt yourself. And stretching is a great way to slow everything down and return back to normal.

On the days in between his visits to torture me, I just do my treadmill and talk to the television to distract my mind from the fact that I have only been walking for five minutes (even though it feels like twenty). This works because when I get caught up in a show, I forget I'm walking. It's true: Time does fly when you're having fun. The other option is sitting and watching not only the program, but my thighs spreading. This way I get to kill two birds with one stone.

As I mentioned before, the other thing I love is my *Wii Fit*! And all the games. You can get a good workout playing tennis, boxing, doing the step exercises, and watching your progress on screen. There is no excuse any longer for not moving that body of yours, so get with the program, any program!

A funny thing happens once you commit to moving that body of yours—you actually begin to like it. I must confess, I think I'm getting a little obsessed. They say it takes three weeks to form a habit. I find that if I don't do something now that I've finally gotten on a roll, my body craves the movement. I feel weird if I don't exercise; for me, it's like not going to church on Sunday. It feels like something is missing from my life. I can feel my body whining, and I've got to get my exercise groove on.

Exercising also makes you stick to your healthy eating plan because you don't want to waste all your hard work on junk. Exercising and bingeing just don't go together. It helps you sleep better at night and regulates your body schedule. Now my body feels the need to be in bed by ten and up between six and seven naturally. I had trouble going to sleep, staying asleep throughout the night, and trouble getting up before. If you have trouble sleeping and find yourself having to take a sleep aid, try exercise. The body knows how to fix these things naturally if we let it.

Last but certainly not least, exercise heightens your self-esteem. I don't know about you, but after I exercise, I feel like I really have done something. I feel better and cuter. I start playing mind games with myself—challenging myself to do more, go longer, and grow even stronger. Again, here it is good to underpromise and overdeliver. If you commit to doing something twenty minutes a day, that will be doable for you. I bet you once you get started, you'll find it hard to stop. High five! I'll meet you on the other side of your new body.

KEEPING IT REAL

- Be honest with your attitude about exercise. Accept the fact that you need to exercise and get rid of the excuses.

- Choose a realistic exercise routine and time for yourself. Enlist a friend or trainer if you have to.

- Make an exercise date with yourself, and stick to it no matter what. We all make time for what is important to us, so make this a high priority.

- Make up a CD or mix on your iPod to help you enjoy your workout.

- Keep a journal on your progress. Challenge yourself to push to the next level every time you meet your goal.

DIVA REFLECTIONS

Once upon a time we exercised naturally—high school dances, tennis, running hither, thither, and yon. We burned calories naturally without thinking about it. Those days are long gone, but the need remains the same. Our bodies still need to move and expend energy. The way they thank us is by burning fat. Our thank-you back is to keep moving so that we stay limber, flexible, fit, and strong. Can you touch your toes without straining? Do you envy babies that eat their feet? Then you need to hit it, sister. This is about more than losing weight. It's about being a better you. Even when my body is screaming for exercise, my mind wages a war against it. Perhaps my mind will evenutually line up and get with the program. But until then, I've decided I will never *want* to exercise because it's not about what I want to do, it's about what I *need*. My body needs to move. It needs to work. It needs to use everything it has to create its own well-being, especially after I sit at a desk all day long writing this to you. I don't know what your day is like or what the demands of your personal world are, but one thing I know, you will not be able to live well without exercise. What you don't use, you will lose. So here's to keeping everything we've got and making it better.

Making Peace with Your Thighs

THERE'S A SAYING, "The Lord loves you just as you are but loves you too much to leave you that way." Truly, we are a work in progress. I think there is a balance between not settling for where you are and appreciating the journey of getting to where you want to be. It can be a fine line sometimes that can either make us descend into paralysis or push us over the edge into overachiever mode. Either way, the balance must be found when it comes to our bodies. Never settle for being out of shape and overweight. However, be realistic as you approach your weight loss. Don't go overboard! There are all sorts of extremes. None of them will serve you well.

First, there is losing weight too fast. Remember that when you do this, you are losing just water at first and then valuable muscle. You don't want to do this. It took you several months or years to get to the size that you are, so give yourself grace to lose it slowly and carefully so that you don't return to the same place with a few extra bags. This is not about a seven-day plan or a six-week plan; this is about the rest of your life. It is about creating habits you can maintain and giving yourself room to fail from time to time. Forgiving yourself is huge because life happens, and when it does, you might reach for something to eat that doesn't serve you well. Enjoy it, get over it, and move on. You should have the leeway to do that as long as it doesn't happen too often.

Losing weight quickly and gaining it back even faster affects your mind-set as well as your body. All that back-and-forth puts a strain on your system and an even greater strain on your self-image. It's too easy to feel like an out-of-control failure every time you repeat this cycle. The more often this occurs, the greater your sense of hopelessness.

Then there is obsessive-compulsive eating, bingeing and purging with laxatives or by inducing vomiting, crossing the line to anorexia and bulimia. This interrupts the natural function of your body and can have serious health complications as weight loss progresses and crosses the line to starvation. Anorexia can affect all areas of the body including the throat, the heart, the gastrointestinal system, and the stomach. It can potentially cause infertility or birth complications. It can also cause rough, scaly skin, brittle nails, depression, kidney stones, the erosion of teeth, enlarged parotid salivary glands . . . shall I go on? Sounds pretty ugly if beauty is what you're after.

I am all for weight reduction surgery in extreme cases, but only if you've gotten counseling and done the right preparation before the surgery. I know many who have had gastric bypass surgery, the band, you name it, but alas, they regained a major portion of the weight because their mind-set toward food was still the same. After losing the weight, they ate to celebrate. I suggest changing your eating habits before the surgery so that you will be able to enjoy the effects of your drastic weight loss without returning to your past sins. Or a more drastic way of putting it: As the Bible states, you won't be like a dog (or a fool) that returns to its vomit.[1] Perhaps if you pictured all that bad food as just that, it would kill your desire for it.

Last but not least, there is another extreme—overdoing the weight loss. I call it the pendulum swing. I always get sad when I see people lose too much weight. I know it's coming back. Your body knows where it is supposed to be as it fights for the amount of weight where it will function at its best and be strong; the person who has lost too much weight gets a false sense of confidence and abdicates the entire idea of maintaining the good habits she learned, rapidly revisiting where she was originally and passing the mark. You should allow for approximately a five-pound fluctuation as your body finds a comfortable place to settle. Keep exercising so those pounds go to the right place instead of just settling around your midsection. This is why I don't like calorie counting or even weighing yourself too much. People get obsessed with a number and forget to look in the mirror.

I've seen many women lose so much weight that it makes their faces look hard and drawn, or worse yet, they end up with massive bags under their eyes. When they add back on a few pounds, their faces fill out and they look beautiful, but they are so busy insisting that they have to weigh 110 that they fail to see that it is not an attractive number for their visage.

So listen to your body and not your taste buds, your heart, or even the "haters" around you. There will be a few who are jealous and tell you that you are too thin because they want you to regain some weight so they can be more comfortable. This is not about them. It is all about you and how you feel in the skin you are in. I have no desire to ever be 103 pounds again. It was a painful time in my existence. I vote for moderation—a slim body with some curve appeal.

Keep in mind that some of the things you are trying to lose on your body have nothing to do with the number on your scale. It may be a matter of focusing on that particular area with exercise to firm, lift, or diminish. This is a healthier approach as opposed to trying to starve it off. Don't hurt yourself! Forget the num-bers—go for the look and the feeling. Don't forsake discipline for a quick fix or take drastic measures. Make peace with where you are, and make purposeful strides toward where you want to go. Don't punish yourself. Reach for the attainable and the sustain-able. Make peace with yourself, and celebrate the body God has given you—one day at a time.

KEEPING IT REAL

- Identify your extreme patterns with eating and/or bingeing.

- Select something that is already hanging in your closet that you would like to get back into (if you haven't done your closet purge yet); otherwise, select a dress size you would like to be, and make that your goal.

- Do not look at your scale more than once a week. Weigh yourself at the same time of day when you do step on that scale.

- Take one day a week off to eat what you want in moderation, preferably before your salad day.

- Write in your food journal why you want to lose weight and how you think it will affect your life. Weed out the fantasies and focus on realistic expectations. (Being skinny is not a guarantee that you'll find love, so will you maintain your healthy lifestyle if you lose the weight but find love eluding you?)

- Write a list of other important priorities besides your weight in order to maintain balance.

DIVA REFLECTIONS

So much is tied to our body image and even how we perceive how others view us that it can send us on a roller-coaster ride of emo-tions where we don't always do the right thing by ourselves. In a world where unrealistic images of what women should look like abound, filling us all with self-loathing, we must remember that the pendulum swings back and forth. (Oh, if only skinny had been in when I was thin as a rail! By the time I got curves, people were over Marilyn Monroe and her other voluptuous cohorts.) The bottom line is that beauty is in the eye of the individual beholder, and as the old folks say, most men like some meat on their bones. No matter what ethnicity, men like curves. Most weight trends are driven by designers pushing their products, fearful that curves will ruin them; that's why I celebrate people like Donna Karan, Norma Kamali, and Michael Kors, who acknowledge and celebrate real women's bodies. According to reports the average woman in America is a size fourteen. Depending on height, bone structure, and build, that could or could not work for you. Instead of aiming for a size two, let's just aim for healthy. Somewhere along the way, our bodies will seek the right place if we do right by them. And that is the gospel truth.

24

Forever and Ever Amen!

EVERY TIME I THINK of the story of Lot's wife, I shudder at the consequences of looking back and clinging to the past.[1] I sometimes wonder, as she scurried up that hill away from the impending doom of the city where she had lived, *What was she thinking when she looked back?* She had been warned not to look back, and yet she did. What did she think she was going to miss? Had she forgotten a favorite article? Was there a friend she hadn't had a chance to say good-bye to in the midst of her hasty retreat? What would make her risk being paralyzed on the spot and missing out on the blessing that was awaiting her once she got past where she was?

Bad habits die hard, don't they? You know what happens when you take a bite of chocolate cake. You lose your mind, and yet that knowledge does not stop you from picking up a piece. "Just a little piece," you say to yourself. Now is the time to complete this renewing of our minds. We have to set healthy boundaries and locate where we cannot revisit. I have to tell you something. There is a man in my life that I refuse to see because if I did, I would be in trouble. The point of this discussion? Know thyself, and behave accordingly. Set boundaries based on the newness of life you want to experience. Don't set yourself up to fall.

For everything that you deny yourself of, find a new alternative to take its place. Fill the vacuum with a new attitude, new activity, or even new snack—out with the old, in with the new!

Don't give in to being stuck. Work through the plateaus in your life. They don't just happen in weight loss; they occur in our relationships, careers, every aspect of life. There will be times when you feel as if you are merely treading water. In those moments, learn how to float. This is the test of longevity—how to handle the moments when nothing is happening. Will you continue to stick to your healthy eating and regime? step it up a notch? or use it as an excuse to look back and to partake of something that you know is going to sabotage the new you? Guard your path with ferocity, and stay on course. Or as my friend Dawn would say, don't get it twisted! This is your body we're talking about! Don't listen to the people that coax you to look back; keep moving forward. You know the conversation, "One piece won't hurt . . ." It might, girlfriend! By now it's not a matter of you *can't* have it (whatever the dish is), it's simply not your preference. Can versus want. Ain't that empowering? Yes!

And let me drop this in your universe. God is on your side on this project, so reach out to Him when you're feeling weak. He wants you to prosper and be in good health even as your soul prospers.[2] He wants you to be a complete woman flourishing spiritually and physically. He knows that how you function and approach life will be driven in a great part based on how you feel as well as how you feel about yourself and Him. When we get the perspective of what a magnificent creation we are, lovingly crafted by the Master Craftsman, we will rise to the responsibility of maintaining our beauty in a way that acknowledges its priceless value.

Remember, you can't have a testimony without a test. You've

got a story to tell other sisters who are still struggling. Make being an inspiration a mind-set you live every day as you maintain your victory. On that note, let me leave you with a few reminders, or should I call them Diva Dos?

Leave emotion out of it. Your weight loss is a decision—You will never feel like doing the right thing or embracing any type of denial. It's just not what human beings do. There will never be a right time to start your new eating plan; there will always be an occasion to indulge your flesh with something that feeds it what it doesn't need. Put your foot down and remember that you are the boss of you. Your lips, your hips, your everything. That being said, pick a date and get started. How about today?

Pray and ask God to forgive you for how you've been treating your body. Then forgive yourself—It's true that it is a crime what we've done to ourselves. But it's never too late to repent and get back on track. Don't hold on to the guilt. Now is not the time to play the victim or beat yourself up; neither gets you what you want—a healthy, strong, slimmed-down body. So let's stay focused. Own your part in the way your body looks. Take responsibility. Power up and do something about it!

Approach your diet prayerfully—Okay, God entrusted your body to you and has let you handle it. Consider what you've done with it. This is a clear indication that you do need help from the One who created your body in the first place to keep it functioning at its best. Ask God to help you every day. He has promised that you will hear a voice giving you clear instruction, saying, "This is the way . . ."[3] I can honestly say I've heard Him tell me, "Don't eat that!" Give your body back to Him, and ask Him to show you how to care for it. After all, He wrote the manual on it! (Complete with instructions on what to eat. Read Leviticus chapter 11 and Deuteronomy chapter 14 in the Bible or *The Maker's Diet* by Jordan Rubin.) We do not necessarily stick to these laws today, although the Jews who maintain a kosher lifestyle do. It is interesting to see what God had to say about certain foods and then see how that lines up with various nutritionists even today.

Learn everything you can about your body and nutrition—You may wonder why I've recommended you read other books. The answer is simple. Knowledge is power. We've all been given portions of truth: Collect it, internalize it, and use it for your benefit. Remember that God has said that understanding is one of the chief things you should pursue.

Pick yourself a pretty journal to chart your progress—Write the vision and make it plain so that you can run with it and stick to it.[4] When something is written, it is binding and established. This is not just an exercise. What you write will hold you accountable. There is the truth in black and white before your eyes. When you know you have to look at what you've done, you'll consider your actions before you leap or bite!

Weigh yourself, measure yourself—Write down that first shocking number, and take a deep breath. This is just the beginning of the journey. Weigh yourself once a week at the same time in the same state. (If you were naked the first time, be naked every time, 'cause clothes weigh something.) Keep in mind that as you build muscle, the numbers may not drop as low as you would like but you are still losing. Measure yourself every two weeks, and of course, your clothes will tell you the truth every time.

Clean out your kitchen cupboards—Girl, get rid of all that expired stuff along with the stuff that isn't good for you at the same time. Don't wait for Niecy Nash to come and help you. If you can't see it, you won't eat it. Don't set yourself up to fail. That's like leaving an alcoholic alone in a bar. My friends say my kitchen is boring because there is no junk; they are right. I call it safe, they call it depressing, but hey! That means they have to eat junk on their own time 'cause I'm over it!

Do a cleanse—Do one physically, mentally, and spiritually. Do a fast to flush out your system. Visit a spa, and get a hydrotherapy colon cleanse. Just start fresh. Take the time to be introspective about the journey you are about to embark on. Remember, turn down your plate and turn up your Bible. You can't live on bread alone.[5] Let God feed you and discover another deeper form of satisfaction. Recalibrate your spirit to focus on becoming a new creature from the inside out.

Do your body calculations, and set your goal—When you know exactly what you're dealing with, you will know how to chart your course and move forward. The truth equips you to make the right choices. Truth helps you to not just make the right choices but to love the choices you make because you know the "why" of what you're doing. This is empowering. Not only does it help you to stay on track; you get to share the information with others who might benefit from what you're learning.

Write your menu for the week—Plan! Plan! Plan! No one gets in a car and says to herself, "Let's just see where it takes me." No! The car goes where you direct it. So decide your dietary direction, and stay on track. This will help when you go to the grocery store so you don't get distracted by all the delicious-looking things that beckon to you from the shelves.

Buy organic or fresh—As much as possible, avoid packages. They are usually packed with sodium, which retains water, and other preservatives that add to the bloat factor. The flavor is found in things that are in their original state. The cleaner you eat, the cleaner your body will remain. It may cost a little more, but what is the price of good health? You'll either pay to eat well up front or pay more for medical treatment later. Do the math.

Start your day with fruit—This gives your body time to wake up and finish its eliminations from the night before. Consider it like brushing your teeth, only you're brushing your colon with good fiber and feeding your body some nutrients at the same time. Have a glass of room-temperature water with fresh lemon—that would be your rinse!

Set your alarm to eat something every three hours—Just in case you are the type to forget. After a while you won't need to do this. If you're eating the right things and being consistent, your body will be its own alarm clock and will tell you it's time to feed it. This keeps your metabolism working and destroying your enemy—fat.

Eat three meals and two to three snacks every day—You've got to keep stoking the fire. That would be your internal engine or metabolism. This will also work to keep you full, never feeling denied. It will automatically remove desperation. You won't feel the need to overeat because you don't know when you will eat again. The body won't feel the need to store fat because it can trust you to feed it again. So full and full of energy—I'm liking that idea.

Stick to the food that is best for your blood type, and be mindful of the foods you are combining—In order to get the optimal health results as you embark on this new way of life, you can do one of two things. You can just follow the plan, or you can choose to up the ante on taking care of yourself to the best of your ability by giving it the best of the best to work with. Choose food that is beneficial to your system while empowering it to function free of extra stress.

Watch your portions—Just because you're cutting down on fat content, sugar, sodium, and calories does not give you permission to double up or double dip. The stomach is really not that large. Most of us have stretched it beyond capacity, thus the onslaught of surgeries to reduce its size. So eat everything on a salad plate. Or eat half of what is on your plate, order appetizer portions when at a restaurant, or ask a friend to split a meal with you when the portions are gargantuan. Remember, you are not living to eat; you eat to live, and you don't need that much to live—just enough to be satisfied comfortably instead of stuffed to the gills. Uncomfortable should be your gauge that you've gone too far.

Drink lots of water!—Research has shown that water helps when trying to lose weight. Those who drank more water lost more weight. Water flushes the system, rehydrates the body, keeps you feeling awake and energetic. There are just too many benefits to drinking water not to do it.

Get your exercise groove on—Get moving, sister. Accept the fact that you are not as active as you once were and you've got to do something about it. So get to dancing, walking, lifting weights, riding a bike, whatever—just do something! You'll feel so much better, and you have everything to lose (fat, that is).

Weigh yourself once a week—Remember, do not hop on the scale every day and freak yourself out. Weight tends to fluctuate and settle, depending on what you ate before you went to bed, when you ate, your activities of the day, etc., so don't pressure yourself every day. You know what you did. Give yourself a week to get results. Chart your results. Yes, write it down! Resist the urge to celebrate and binge when you've lost. Make goals for yourself, and celebrate in moderation when you reach a weight goal marker, like say every ten pounds.

Take a day off from exercise once a week—Even God took a rest, and so should you. Don't be a slave to the gym; you will come to resent it. You need a day to revive your engines and gain new strength for the week ahead. So pick a day, the best day for you, and celebrate giving yourself and your body a break. After all your hard work, you deserve it.

Eat anything you want once a week—Again, if you ever slip into denial mode, you are going to binge, and we might never see you again. So let your psyche know you can still eat whatever you want—once a week (that would be on the same day). Don't overdo it; just have enough to satisfy your taste buds. Over time your choices will change as you get used to feeling good by eating what is good for you, or at least I hope they will.

Locate new favorite "treats"—Every vacuum needs to be filled with something, or it will leave the door open to things that are not conducive to your victory. So experiment with new, healthy "junk foods." Instead of potato chips that are fried, try some that are baked. Try rice cakes. I love jicama sticks dipped in hummus. Find new delights to treat yourself with. I make my own tabouli that is yummmm-my! (I'll give you the recipe later.)

Keep a daily journal of what you are eating and doing—This is important. You will be able to track your progress and know where you need to make changes to your program. This will also keep you in touch with how you are feeling. Mood will sometimes have a lot to do with what you eat and when. Track the following things in your journal:

- Date
- Time you got up
- Breakfast
- Snack
- Lunch
- Snack
- Dinner
- Snack
- Water (how much)
- Exercise (what you did, how long)
- Beverages
- Mood
- Affirmation (or Scripture) of the day
- Something to be grateful for
- Time you went to bed
- A funny story or thought

Get plenty of sleep—Speaking of sleeping, you need to get your rest. The body does not lose weight well when it is stressed out and tired. The average body needs at least seven to eight hours of sleep. Try to regulate your schedule as much a possible. TiVo your late-night shows, and watch them later. Hey, those guys all tape during the day and are asleep while you're up watching them—what's wrong with this picture? No one is worth losing sleep over, especially if you're trying to lose weight.

Get an accountability partner—If you're not calling Jenny, call somebody. Find someone to partner with on your new lease on eating. My sister is my partner. I'm trying to get my brother to join us. You can put your journals on your computer and just e-mail them back and forth to one another. When you know you have to tell someone what you're doing, it keeps you in line. At this point I say whatever works, do it!

Feed your spirit more than you feed your body—When your spirit is full, your body can't be the boss of you because you're already full. When your spirit is strong and you're listening more for the voice of God, the voice of your body can't drown out all the good stuff you are already hearing. Is it starve a fever, feed a cold or the other way around? In this case, it's about feeding what will really sustain you and strengthen you to withstand all distractions and self-defeating temptations.

Decide what you want more—Leverage is key in all decisions. What is more important to you? The taste of that cupcake or the pleasure of another pound gone at the end of the week; those greasy chips or a lower cholesterol level and good health; eating for the pleasure of it or being around to see your children grow up and marry? Lamentations 1:9, ESV, says, "She took no thought of her future; therefore her fall is terrible." If you don't consider the future of your choices, shortsightedness and the need for instant gratification can have unpleasant, lasting effects and damaging consequences. It's all about perspective, big-picture thinking, and choices—so make the right ones.

Maintain a grateful spirit—Joy is a gift from God that gives us strength. Depression will rob you of your perspective and keep you from seeing the blessings at hand. When you are downcast, you are rendered weak and powerless. This will also affect your willpower. So, out with the negative, dwell on the positive—things that are true, honest, just, whatever things are pure, lovely, of good report, if there is any virtue, any praise, think on these things.[6] These things will lift you, keep hope alive, and give you the strength to go forward another day—to say no to your wants and yes to your needs. Rejoice in the disciplines that make you strong and give you longevity. Praise God for your health and all that He affords to keep you being the best you can be. It's all a gift, my sister, which means the Giver doesn't have to give it, and yet He did. So give thanks—at the beginning of the day, before every meal, before you lie down to sleep. Give thanks.

a few recipes to boot

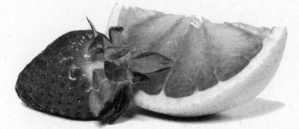

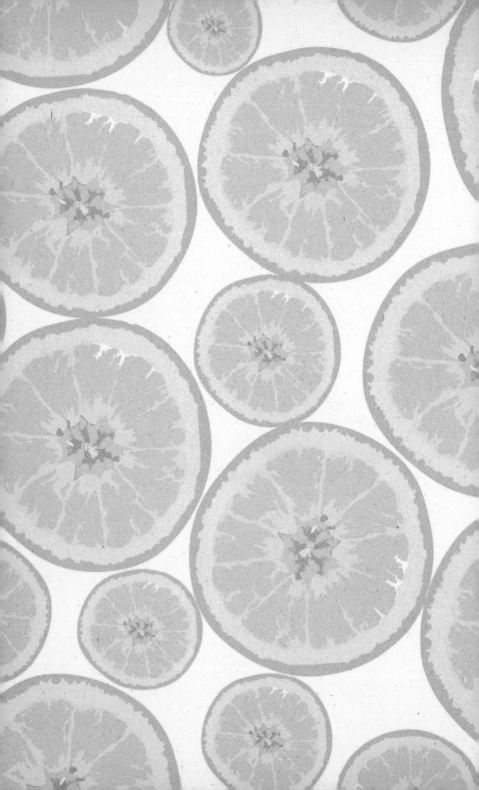

These are just a few of the things that I fix for myself that are my staples, or should I say my "converted treats" or fillers that are nutritious but also delicious.

Apple Smoothie
- ½ cup of nonfat Greek yogurt
- ½ cup of skim milk or almond milk
- 1 apple
- 6 cubes of ice
- 2 scoops of protein powder

Blend on high.

Caribbean Smoothie
- ½ cup coconut water
- 1 cup of mango slices
- ½ cup of nonfat Greek yogurt
- 1 cup ice
- 2 scoops of protein powder

Blend on high.

Peanut Smoothie
- 1 tablespoon fresh, unsalted peanut butter (or almond, depending on your blood type)
- ½ cup nonfat yogurt
- ½ cup skim milk
- 2 scoops protein powder
- 1 cup ice

Blend on high.

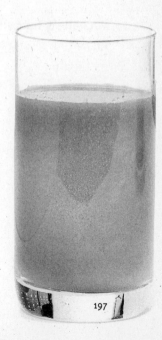

Coffee Smoothie

- ½ cup nonfat yogurt
- ½ cup skim, soy, or almond milk
- 2 scoops vanilla-flavored protein powder
- 6 cubes of ice
- 1 tablespoon coffee

Blend on high. If you would like a thicker smoothie, make a cup of coffee and freeze it the night before. In the morning, put the coffee ice in with the other ingredients and blend. Yum!

Fruit-Flavored Water

- ½ watermelon
- 2 cups of ice
- cold water

Place these ingredients in a pitcher together. Let it sit for an hour. The fruit will naturally flavor the water. It is delicious and refreshing. You can also try this with cantaloupe, honeydew, cucumbers, oranges, or strawberries.

Michelle's Tabouli

- 1 handful of spinach
- 1 carrot
- 1 small handful of almonds or walnuts
- 2 figs
- 1 green apple (don't tell the FFL people!)

Place in a food processor or blender and let it fly until chopped! Delicious!

Fruit Salad

- 1 mango
- ½ pineapple
- 1 papaya
- ¼ small watermelon
- 1 apple
- seeds from one small pomegranate

Place in a bowl overnight. The flavors begin to saturate one another. You can double the recipe and make enough to last a few days.

Garbage Salad

- ½ cucumber
- ½ package of mushrooms
- shredded carrots
- ½ red bell pepper
- ½ yellow bell pepper
- 1 avocado
- 2 hard-boiled eggs
- sweet grape tomatoes
- ½ cup of canned garbanzo beans or chickpeas, rinsed

Toss all ingredients in a bowl together. Enjoy with your favorite low-fat dressing or sprinkle herbs over your salad along with a little olive oil. Yummy and filling!

Sweet Potato Fries

- 2 sweet potatoes, peeled and cut in strips ½-inch wide
- olive oil
- sea or kosher salt
- Italian herbs or seasoned salt

Preheat oven to 400° F. Spray or wipe a thin layer of cooking oil on your cookie sheet. Lay potato strips on cookie sheet. Brush on olive oil. Sprinkle with salt and herbs. Bake approximately 30 to 40 minutes. For even browning, turn them every 10 minutes.

A variation on this for sweet potatoes is to cut thin slices of two sweet potatoes. Toss in a Ziploc bag with olive oil, a dash of sea salt, and some rosemary. Place in a dish and microwave for 5 minutes on high or until tender. You can add a splash of agave for the sweet.

Light and Delicious Soup

- 1 chicken, cut up
- 2 medium, sweet yellow onions
- 3 tomatoes
- 1 hot red pepper (I prefer dried)
- 1 small can of tomato paste
- 1 cup of chicken boullion

Brown chicken in a pot. Steam tomatoes and onion together in a separate pot. When they are soft, put in blender with pepper. Liquefy tomatoes, pepper, and onions; pour over chicken. Add 2 to 3 cups of water. Simmer 30 to 40 minutes. Add tomato paste and bouillion. This is comfort food!

Nancy's Zero-Cal Soup

- ⅔ cup sliced carrots
- ¼ cup chopped onion
- 2 cloves of garlic, chopped

Spray cooking spray on pan, and sauté all of the above.

Add:
- 3 cups fat-free bouillon
- 1½ cups of cabbage, shredded
- ½ cup green beans
- 1 tablespoon tomato paste
- A dash of basil, oregano, and salt

Cover and cook approximately 15 minutes.

Stir in:
- ½ cup diced zucchini

Cook an additional 3 to 4 minutes.

This is the base. You can add things like black beans or your favorite frozen vegetable to the mix. Add about 2 cups of chicken stock for some extra flavor along with some red pepper flakes or low-sodium soy sauce, whatever your taste.

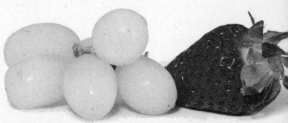

Stir-Fried Cabbage

- 2 strips of bacon or 2 slices of Canadian bacon
- 1 head of cabbage, cut in strips
- 1 small sweet yellow onion, sliced
- 2 teaspoons sugar
- black pepper

Place bacon in pan and cook 'til soft. Take bacon out and discard; we just want the grease. Place cabbage and onion slices in pot. Sprinkle sugar on top, and sprinkle with black pepper. Place lid on pot and allow to simmer until cabbage is soft. Stir after the cabbage and onion begin to get soft. This is a guilty pleasure!

Pumpkin Soup

- 8 ounces mushrooms, chopped
- ½ cup onions, chopped
- 2 tablespoons unsalted butter
- 1 tablespoon curry powder
- 2 tablespoons flour
- 3 cups chicken stock
- 16 oz. canned pumpkin
- 1 tablespoon honey
- 1 cup low-fat yogurt
- Add nutmeg, salt, and pepper to taste

Cook mushrooms and onions in butter until soft. Add curry powder and flour and stir over heat for 5 minutes. Remove from the heat and place in a stockpot. Add chicken stock, pumpkin, honey, and nutmeg. Place mixture in blender to completely blend; do in several small batches. Add salt and pepper to taste and simmer about 15 minutes. Add yogurt and simmer on very low heat, but do not boil.

Chef Devin's Roasted Vegetable Soup

- 3 cups chicken broth
- ¼ cup diced red potatoes
- 2 tablespoons diced celery
- 2 tablespoons diced onions
- ⅓ cup diced tomatoes
- ¼ cup chopped butternut squash
- ¼ cup chopped zucchini
- ¼ cup tomato sauce
- ¼ cup low-fat Greek yogurt
- 1 tablespoon brown sugar

Simmer together in a separate pot:

- 2 tablespoons butter, melted
- 2 tablespoons flour

Bring chicken broth to a boil. Add vegetables and cook 10-15 minutes until vegetables are tender. Add tomato sauce, simmer for 5 minutes. Add yogurt, cook 2 minutes, then thicken with flour/ butter mixture. Let everything simmer for a minute. Add brown sugar to lift flavor.

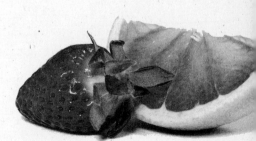

Easy Chicken Salad

- 1 chicken breast, cubed
- ¼ sweet yellow onion
- 1 teaspoon mustard
- 1 celery stalk, chopped
- dash of salt and pepper
- ½ cup low-fat yogurt

Mix together and put on top of lettuce. Add a few slices of avocado.

Easy Dressing

- Puree a sweet tomato in the blender.
- Add 2 tablespoons of olive oil, a dash of rosemary, an herbal salt mixture, and a squirt of agave or a packet of Equal or Splenda, if you must.

You can substitute raspberries or mandarin orange slices for the tomato and get the same yummy dressing. Chop up some nuts and add for a bit of the crunch factor.

notes

Introduction
1. See Genesis 3.

Chapter 1: Looking in the Mirror
1. See John 8:32.

Chapter 2: The Real Issue
1. See Mark 5:21-34.

Chapter 3: Naked and Ashamed
1. See Genesis 2 and 3.
2. See Luke 12:48.

Chapter 4: A Shadow of My Former Self
1. See Daniel 1:11-15.

Chapter 5: Putting Away Childish Things
1. See Matthew 26:41.
2. 1 Corinthians 13:11, NIV

Chapter 7: Attitude Check
1. See Luke 11:17.

Chapter 8: From Your Lips to Your Hips
1. See Philippians 4:8.

Chapter 9: What Have You Got to Lose?
1. See Isaiah 61:3, KJV.
2. See Ecclesiastes 9:11.

Chapter 10: Going Nowhere Fast
1. See Galatians 6:7.
2. webmd.com/diet/features/the-cabbage-soup-diet
3. webmd.com/diet/features/the-rice-diet-solution
4. Lemonadedietrecipe.org

Chapter 11: The Truth about Fasting
1. See Mark 9:28-29.

Chapter 12: Extreme Makeovers
1. See John 4:7-29.

Chapter 14: Eenie, Meenie, Minie, Yo-Yo!

1. See Genesis 1:29.

Chapter 15: What's Really Eating You?

1. See 1 Peter 5:7.
2. See Psalm 46:10.

Chapter 16: Empty Calories and Other Unnecessary Evils

1. Proverbs 13:12, NLT
2. See Hebrews 12:1.

Chapter 17: Apples, Pears, and Other Body Types

1. See Proverbs 4:7.

Chapter 18: Finding the Perfect Combination

1. Harvey and Marilyn Diamond, *Fit for Life* (New York: Warner, 1985), 162.
2. See Psalm 139:14.

Chapter 19: The Right Foundation

1. David Zinczenko with Ted Spiker, *The Abs Diet for Women* (New York: Rodale, 2007), 29.
2. Ibid., 4.
3. See Hosea 4:6, NIV.

Chapter 20: The Ultimate Love Affair

1. Matthew 19:19, NLT
2. See Psalm 139:13.

Chapter 21: All Things Are Lawful

1. See John 8:32.
2. Harvey and Marilyn Diamond, *Fit for Life* (New York: Warner, 1985), 139–190.

Chapter 23: Making Peace with Your Thighs

1. See Proverbs 26:11.

Chapter 24: Forever and Ever Amen!

1. See Genesis 19:6-26.
2. See 3 John 1:2.
3. See Isaiah 30:21.
4. See Habakkuk 2:2.
5. See Matthew 4:4.
6. See Philippians 4:8.

recommended reading

Fit for Life
BY HARVEY AND MARILYN DIAMOND

The Abs Diet for Women
BY DAVID ZINCZENKO WITH TED SPIKER

Eat Right for Your Type
BY DR. PETER J. D'ADAMO

Blood Types, Body Types and You
BY JOSEPH CHRISTIANO

The Answer is in Your Bloodtype
BY STEVEN M. WEISSBERG, M.D, & JOSEPH CHRISTIANO

Eat This, Not That
BY DAVID ZINCZENKO WITH MATT GOULDING

Busy People's Low-fat Cookbook
BY DAWN HALL

The Cooking Cardiologist
BY RICHARD COLLINS, M.D.

The Four Day Diet
BY DR. IAN SMITH

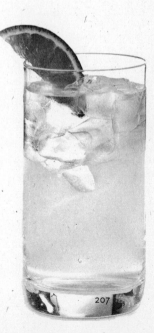

about the author

AS A BEST-SELLING AUTHOR, speaker, singer, and inspiration to audiences all over the world, Michelle McKinney Hammond pinpoints the root causes of relational issues while sharing life-changing insights for "living, loving, and overcoming." It's Michelle's combination of grace, truth, transparency, and humor that has landed her in numerous media outlets, including *Essence* and *Ebony* magazines, the *Chicago Tribune,* and the *New York Times,* which called Michelle "the most visible face of the evangelical advice industry for single men and women."

Michelle has written thirty-four books and sold more than two million copies worldwide. She also cohosted for ten years the Emmy Award–winning women's talk show *Aspiring Women.* Her numerous television appearances include *The Morning Show with Mike and Juliet* on Fox, *Politically Incorrect* with Bill Maher on ABC, *The Other Half* on NBC, *Baisden After Dark* on TV One, *Oh Drama!* on BET, *Soap Talk* on SOAPnet, *The 700 Club, The Morris Cerullo Show, Life Today with James Robison,* as well as appearances on Fox Chicago and *WGN Morning News* as the featured relationships expert.

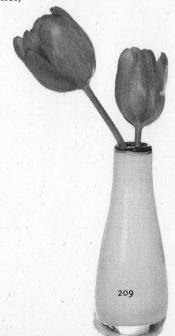